Neurologic Evaluation of the Newborn and the Infant

Neurologic Evaluation of the Newborn and the Infant

Claudine Amiel-Tison, M.D.
Associate Professor
Port-Royal Hôpital, Paris

Albert Grenier, M.D.
Former Chef de Clinique of the Faculté de Paris
Chief of Service, Department of Pediatrics
Hôpital de Bayonne, France

English translation and adaptation by

Jean J. Steichen, M.D.
Associate Professor of Pediatrics
Obstetrics and Gynecology
University of Cincinnati, Department
of Pediatrics/Newborn Division
The Children's Hospital Medical Center
and the Children's Hospital Research
Foundation, Cincinnati, Ohio

Paula Steichen-Asch, Ph.D.
Adjunct Assistant Professor of Psychology
University of Cincinnati
Department of Psychology and Psychiatry
Cincinnati, Ohio

Colleen Paxton Braun, Ed.D.
University of Cincinnati Medical Center
Cincinnati, Ohio

Distributed by
YEAR BOOK MEDICAL PUBLISHERS • INC.
35 EAST WACKER DRIVE, CHICAGO

eiro

Translated from *Coupes anatomiques du nouveau-né* by Claudine Amiel-Tison, M.D., and Albert Grenier, M.D. Copyright by Masson, Paris, 1980.

Library of Congress Cataloging in Publication Data

Main entry under title:

Amiel-Tison, Claudine.
Neurologic evaluation of the newborn and the infant.

Translation of: Coupes anatomiques du nouveau-né.
Bibliography: p.
Includes index.
1. Infants (Newborn)—Medical examinations.
2. Pediatric neurology—Diagnosis. I. Grenier, Albert. II. Steichen, Jean J. III. Braun, Colleen Paxton. IV. Title. [DNLM: 1. Neurologic examination—In infancy and childhood. 2. Infant, Newborn. WS 340 A516na]
RJ255.5.A4713 618.92′80475 82-62
ISBN 0-89352-164-7 AACR2

ISBN 0-89352-164-7

Library of Congress Catalog Card Number: 82-62

Printed in the United States of America

Preface to the English Edition

Twenty years ago, I began a prospective follow-up of some of the infants treated in our Intensive Care Nursery. I was particularly interested in whether changes in the traditional modes of therapy, which my colleagues and I were following, were associated with an increase or a decrease in abnormalities of the developing nervous system. From the beginning of neonatology, the need for the early detection of signs which would predict later intellectual or neurological dysfunction was seen as an imperative. Any evaluations were hampered, however, by the lack of a standardized method for examination of the nervous system in the first year of life. The Bayley and Gessell tests of infant development had standardized motor scales, but they did not provide enough information to permit identification of the type of and the mechanism for delays in the development of neuromotor function. Eight years ago, Dr. Amiel-Tison resolved this problem. Drawing on the works of her French colleagues, particularly Drs. Andre-Thomas, Ajuriaguerra, and Saint-Anne Dargassies, and her own rich clinical experience, Dr. Amiel-Tison created a simple system for the comprehensive assessment of the changing neuromotor function during the first year of life. She suggested that two people participate in the examination, one to perform the maneuvers and the other to observe and record. As her assistant, I was able to work with Dr. Amiel-Tison on many occasions. I learned to evaluate neuromotor function in the infant using her method, and this has become an indispensable part of our neonatal follow-up program. A complete description of this method has, until now, only been available in French. Now, we have this excellent, easily understood translation which, fortunately, still contains some of the author's Gallic turn of phrase.

It is not an easy task to describe normal neuromotor function in an infant during the first year of life. Each month has its own norm. The flexors of the hips and legs in an infant at birth, born after a 40-week gestation, are hypertonic. The same muscle groups are much more relaxed at 6 months of age. The method of examination outlined in this book assesses passive tone at monthly intervals. This identifies abnormalities in the pattern of waxing and waning of muscle tone, which occurs from late fetal life to 1 year of age. It also permits identification of asymmetries of tone. Active tone is also evaluated at monthly intervals, which considers postural activity in response to changes in body position. The tests of both passive and active muscle tone and activity are placed on a grid. This grid displays the observed response next to the expected performance for each age. Each observation in the method is clearly, carefully, and completely described and any problems noted.

This book also includes many helpful clinical hints, such as the prognostic importance of finding a *straightening reaction* at 7 months of age in the absence of sitting. With this system we have identified many types of neuromotor dysfunction early in the first year of life, and have been able to document their course. Some of these abnormalities disappear, while others evolve into classical patterns of disease.

In addition, the author also stresses the importance of the *lateral abduction reaction*, which was not included in earlier descriptions of her method. This maneuver often provides an early clue that cerebral palsy may be developing. A normal lateral abduction reaction at 3 months of age in 384 infants correctly predicted normal neuromotor integrity and subsequent neuromotor function. On the other hand, 18 of 35 infants with an abnormal reaction at 3 months of age developed cerebral palsy. It appears, therefore, that with this test cerebral palsy can be predicted at an early age and active intervention can be undertaken if desired. It is discouraging, however, to learn that in the author's experience those subjects enrolled in physical therapy programs at an early age did no better than those for whom physical therapy was started at a later age.

The successful examiner of the young infant must be a patient and careful observer. This is particularly true if the liberated *motor activity following manual immobilization of the head* is to be elicited. This new test of neuromotor function holds great promise of providing the early diagnostic tool desired by neonatologists. In the first 2 months of life, latent motor development can be manifested by stabilizing the head for 5 minutes and then proceeding with a complex series of maneuvers. The artfulness and skill required for this test will be difficult for some, but it is worth the effort, particularly, if after 5 minutes the infant looks at the examiner "as if charmed". Who can resist being a charmer?

Dr. Amiel-Tison has provided us with an approach to the examination of the neuromotor system in the young infant. Her book will be required reading for those following the progress of newborn infants born at risk of having neurological or developmental abnormalities.

William H. Tooley, M.D.
Professor of Pediatrics
University of California

Preface to the French Edition

The neurological evaluation of the immature child must be interpreted within a chronological and developmental framework. Accordingly, the approach to the neurological assessment of the child should differ from that applied to an adult. The examiner must understand the evolution of the child in order to interpret maturation and successive functional organizational levels (i.e., the evaluation must encompass both diachronic and synchronic perspectives).

Neurological diagnosis is based on a clinical evaluation of various signs, symptoms, and reactions, some of which are diagnostic of central nervous system abnormality. This procedure is complicated in the pediatric patient. The child's responses during the examination may be considered normal or abnormal, depending on age at the time of evaluation. Symptomatology is ascribed 1) according to the presence or absence of primary (i.e., archaic) reflexes, and 2) the appearance of certain functions manifest in a linear progression during ontogeny.

Likewise, linearity of the evolution of man must be understood as it is manifest. Evolution may be represented in the persistence of certain features, or the appearance or disappearance of others. This process may unfold within a particular subsystem or involve the complete organizational structure. One must note the integrational level at the time any specific sign appears. Some functions present at birth may be extinguished for a time, only to reappear later. Disassociation within the same functional system may be evident, e.g., hypertonic axial muscles concurrent with hypotonia in the muscles of the extremities. During evolution, axial muscle tone increases while the tone in the extremities decreases. Symptoms, signs, and reflexes must be studied and integrated within an organizational framework. For example, unique evolutionary properties are observed in the sitting posture or walking. Modification of tone, straightening reflexes, and equilibrium evolve simultaneously.

Child development can be studied by referring to standard developmental curves or by applying specific methods of the neurological examination. These methodologies are complementary.

Standardized curves for early infancy were first established by Izar and Simon; however, Gesell *et al.* defined certain evolutionary progressions based on extensive observations of infant development. Gesell has always held that his studies were not designed to establish an intelligence test allowing calculations of developmental scores. Similarly, Buhler has established developmental curves and tests for the young infant, insisting that these curves should be analyzed at different ages. In France, the most commonly used developmental curves for infants between 4 and 30 months of age are those established by Brunet-Lezine. The curves developed by Casati-Lezine and adapted from Piaget are used for infants between 6 months and 2 years of age.

When these tests and curves are used as measurement instruments, testing difficulties and general characteristics of the child must be taken into consideration. Results serve as indicators of direction and orientation, rather than absolute values. Abnormal findings and handicaps must be confirmed by more precise methodologies; however, the limitations of these approaches must be recognized as well. Wallon's preface to the work of Brunet and Lezine stressed that progressive developmental curves and developmental stages according to age do not establish an absolute norm for progress in any one child. Rather, precise delineation of developmental steps facilitates identification of normal variations in individual development in order to establish the significance of these individual variations. More precise studies and clinical observations must be undertaken.

Over the last several decades, great progress has been made in the neurological evaluation of the newborn infant. Research has included studies of spontaneous and evoked movements, changes in posture and equilibrium, new and archaic reflexes and reactions, and the study of social and sensory development. Recent studies have shown that sensory development occurs much earlier than believed previously. Works by Pratt, Peiper, Prechtl, Beintema, Lefevre, Diament, Illingworth, and others have contributed to this research. McGraw and Halverson have focused on specific aspects of the evolutional process. In France, these studies have been expanded by Andre-Thomas. With the help of his collaborators, especially Saint-Anne Dargassies, he has opened numerous new avenues to the understanding of clinical neurology. Koupernik and Dailly have made important contributions as well.

Neurological evaluation of the infant must be viewed from a diagnostic and prognostic perspective, as understood by Claudine Amiel-Tison and Albert Grenier. While there seems to be an abundance of literature describing neurologic symptomatology, few instruments assess the evolution of the child (especially the premature child or the infant at risk) or establish a neurological profile according to age. The most crucial periods for carrying out such an assessment are birth and 2, 7, and 12 months, corrected age. A summary of this kind establishes more clearly the importance of certain early neurological disorders. This is especially apparent with regard to the hyperkinetic child (i.e., the old French school classification of "motor instability").

A grid has been established by Claudine Amiel-Tison for the neurological evaluation of the child during the first year of life ("A method for neurological evaluation within the first year of life," *Current Problems in Pediatrics,* Volume 7, No. 1, 1976). This grid more precisely describes the broadly defined syndrome of minimal brain damage detailed in the works of Strauss and Lehtinen. In this syndrome, there is a general disorganization of cognitive proprioceptive motor and affective development. The term "minimal brain damage" was rejected in 1962 by the International Study Group of Oxford in order to avoid a pathogenic connotation. The term "minimal cerebral dysfunction" was favored. Studies of minimal cerebral dysfunction have evidenced significant methodological deficiencies, as shown by Touwen and Prechtl. There is no substitute for controlled and prospective longitudinal studies.

As the clinical neurological symptomatology of the young child is extremely rich, some neurological disorders may be found in all infants at risk. It is important to know the extent of these disorders and to determine whether they are transient or permanent. Every infant at risk may show certain atypical symptoms that, if overestimated, could be considered prognostic of cerebral palsy. In this work, we will find an approach lacking in other reports. Specific maneuvers are described. These maneuvers result in typical reactions which, if present, are characteristic of normal motor function. An example is the lateral abduction reaction, known as Grenier's maneuver. The characteristic response to this maneuver eliminates the possibility of cerebral palsy. Grenier has also described an induction maneuver that can contribute to an improvement of postural regulation and correction of fixed postures or abnormal motor activity. While the presence of this reaction is highly significant, its absence has no specific prognostic value. For a long time, authors have insisted on the importance of neck movements and tonic modifications. Grenier has shown that certain obligatory and stereotypic motor activities can be suppressed by manual fixation of the neck. When maintained in this position, the child seems to engage in communication with the examiner. Wakefulness is increased, the basic tone is modified, movements become smoother and better coordinated, and axial hypotonia is decreased. The possibility to liberate the motor activity by modifying the child's posture must not simply remain a simple observation, but should be used during physical therapy.

Even so, the diagnosis is an essential element of the neurological examination. It is the prognosis that remains foremost on the mind of the family, as well as the physician. In this work, many precautions and pitfalls that must be avoided before formulating an abnormal prognosis are pointed out. The authors also call our attention to the importance to take the elasticity of the infant's brain into consideration. This work is intended to describe and evaluate signs and syndromes present at a given time and to describe with caution the evolution of these signs within the evolutionary framework of any given child.

Julien de Ajuriaguerra, M.D.
Collège de France

Introduction

Advancements in neonatal technology and early neurologic intervention have fostered the recent interest in the neurologic evaluation of the infant and newborn. Survival of a growing percentage of high-risk neonates–those most likely to suffer neurologic sequelae–has been accomplished through the specialized care provided in the intensive care nursery. Still, hospitalization during this difficult period of weeks or months may be marked by such medical complications as multiple pneumothoraces, ligation of patent ductus arteriosis, and chronic pulmonary problems following artificial ventilation.

Examiners sensitive to these early difficulties may expect that evidence of cerebral damage and cerebral palsy will be revealed in the course of routine examinations. However, there is a growing awareness that it is not uncommon for premature infants–even those born at 1000 grams–to evidence age-appropriate neurologic maturation at term date (e.g., normal interactional patterns, pursuit of light, motor performance, and primary reflexes). This favorable outcome has become more routine as the result of both a) greater success in preventing intrapartum asphyxia, and b) more proficient neonatal and postnatal management of the newborn.

Because results of the evaluation carried out prior to discharge from the neonatal-perinatal center are not predictive of subsequent outcome, infants-at-risk must undergo repeated examinations at regular intervals during the first year of life. Appropriate evaluative tools would integrate customary methods of neuromotor evaluation and psychomotor testing.

A summary review of recent literature[12,20,24,30] underscores three important findings relative to the neurologic outcome of the high-risk infant:

1. Motor handicaps and cerebral damage can be diagnosed as early as the third and fourth month of life; however, the incidence of these disorders is rare.
2. Prior to initiating intervention appropriate for severe disorders, specific methods should be applied in order to isolate the problem and

confirm a diagnosis. Transient neuromotor abnormalities, which may be attributable to minor neurologic lesions, are not uncommon during the first year of life and often become most pronounced between six and eight months corrected postnatal age. Those abnormalities stemming from minor lesions generally disappear with maturation of the central nervous system. Detection of such abnormalities would hold no prognostic interest were it not for the evolving correlation between these findings and subsequent learning disabilities. Transient lesions appear to be coupled with underlying cellular injury manifest at some subsequent developmental stage as problems in language development, behavorial disorders, fine motor deficiencies, and decreased intellectual functioning. This casual association justifies the assignment of primary prognostic importance to those neurologic abnormalities discovered during routine evaluation in the first year of life.

3. Although it is difficult to determine which abnormalities may foster ongoing sequelae, a motor prognosis in the first few weeks of life appears to be indispensable.

Still, classical methods of neuromotor evaluation yield little useful information prior to four months of age. New approaches to evaluation of the neuromotor system have been designed to overcome deficiencies in existing evaluative instruments. By exploring in greater depth the active muscle tone, the newborn's motor coordination potential is assessed through a series of precise stimulations evoking specific motor movements. These manipulations–especially those detecting the presence of lateral abduction reaction of the hip–enable, if present, early determination of normal function. The reaction will be discussed in great detail in Chapter 4.

In carrying out a neurologic evaluation of the high-risk infant, several points should be taken into consideration. First, it is incorrect to assume that the high-risk infant will necessarily develop severe motor handicaps. In actuality, it is important to minimize the number of infants suspected to have cerebral palsy. Second, the level of motor functioning should be assessed as early as the first weeks of life–repeated monthly examinations are necessary in order to detect transient abnormalities during the first 12 months.

1. The level of surveillance may be relaxed if these abnormalities disappear by the end of the first year.
2. However, should the anomalies persist, follow-up would be warranted until normalization is realized.
3. Finally, medical and educational support should be directed toward those infants evidencing abnormalities associated with increased risk of subsequent handicaps.

Recent diagnostic innovations–notably the CAT scanner–have yielded major advancements in the evaluation of perinatal-cerebral lesions; yet, minor damage can either escape detection or be overestimated. Accordingly, the clinical approach can be viewed as integral to the objectives of the neurologic examination and follow-up. Such objectives should encompass identification of those infants at risk on the basis of neuromotor anomalies–including even transient abnormalities–appearing during the first year of life. The organic basis for potential intellectual or behavioral deficits could then be delineated within this broad classification of minimal brain dysfunction.

The proposed protocol for clinical diagnosis is not exhaustive; rather, it encompasses only those neurologic examinations of current research interest. The following chapters will describe each of the proposed techniques, analyze the varying response patterns, and discuss alternate interpretations of these components. A basis for long-term prognosis is proposed by Claudine Amiel-Tison in a table of the most frequently observed first year anomalies (see page 52). Also included (see Chapter 5) is a neuromotor examination developed by Albert Grenier to confirm the integrity of neuromotor potential during the first weeks of life, a period during which definitive assessments have not been possible. In this examination, the infant's alertness and transformation of motor aptitude are assessed through a maneuver entailing manual fixation of the neck. The nature of the infant's response can confirm a prognosis for neuromotor integrity despite apparent pathology, thus providing a basis for eliminating diagnosis of cerebral palsy.

Although the procedure lacks current clinical application, the methodology and theoretical interpretations will be discussed.

Claudine Amiel-Tison, M.D.
Albert Grenier, M.D.

Acknowledgments

We thank Annette Tison for her valuable and talented help. Her drawings have depicted the movements of the newborn with such precision and perfection that we were often stimulated to review our somewhat vague observations and descriptions of these maneuvers.

Our very special thanks go to the personnel of the Reeducation Center for Handicapped Children "Aintzina" of Bayonne and most especially to Dr. L. Hurmic, Dr. P. H. Vima, and M. C. Solomiac, occupational therapist. They have been our long-time collaborators and have given us invaluable help in developing the additional neuromotor examination. The clinical applications of this maneuver are described in this text.

Mrs. J. Balais-Solomiac, occupational and physical therapist in the neonatal service of the Bayonne Medical Center, has contributed to this work. Her contact with the children and her most acute sense and understanding of motor activity in the very young infant has laid the groundwork for this study. She also had the rather monumental task of taking the numerous photographs. Without these photographs this work would not have been possible. We are most deeply indebted to her for her contributions.

The photographs illustrating the maneuvers in the examination grid were initially published in the *Concours Medical* 21:3501, 1979. We thank Dr. Vigy and Dr. Koupernik for giving us permission to reproduce these photographs. We express our special gratitude to Ms. Nancy McKenney for her expert help in preparing the English edition of this work.

Contents

Preface to the English Edition v

Preface to the French Edition vii

Introduction xi

Acknowledgments xiv

1. Definitions of Tone and Posture 1

2. Preliminary Aspects of the Neuromotor Examination 5

3. Normal Development During the First Year of Life: Identification of Anomalies and Use of the Grid 11

4. Additional Neuromotor Examination: Lateral Abduction Reaction of the Lower Limb Obtained by a Hemilateral Progressive Motor Reaction (Directed Motor Activity) 57

5. Expression of Liberated Motor Activity (LMA) Following Manual Immobilization of the Head 87

Appendices 111

References 127

Index 131

Chapter 1

Definitions of Tone and Posture

Although numerous neurophysiological studies over the last 30 years have generated a wealth of information contributing to the understanding of muscle tone, we believe that those aspects of the physical evaluation described by André-Thomas et al.[34] remain integral to the clinical examination. Accordingly, the terminology used in this volume is consistent with the definitions reported by André-Thomas and De Ajuriaguerra.[34] Because we preface our discussion of muscle tone with only a brief review of terminology, we suggest that the reader refer to the definitions included in the original studies.[28,29,35]

At this point we shall not elaborate on the so-called *primary reflexes*, as a detailed review is included in the actual description of our examination and the corresponding grid. We remind the reader that a certain number of reflexes can be recognized as early as the first few days of life. These primary reflexes are the hallmark of a particular developmental stage and disappear over the following months. Although the presence of these primary reflexes can be considered an indication of the integrity of the central nervous system (CNS) during the first few weeks of life, their progressive disappearance is consistent with normal development. Reflex manifestation remains highly tone dependent.

PASSIVE TONE

We propose the study of passive tone as a means of identifying transient anomalies. The description of each maneuver, as reexamined in the grid, corresponds to classic interpretation. Detection of anomalies in passive tone is accomplished through the study of extensibility and flapping. Muscle extensibility, examined segment by segment, consists of maneuvers that evaluate the amplitude of a slow movement applied to an infant in a passive state. Most commonly, the results are expressed as an angle that is estimated, but not measured, by the examiner. In other instances, passive tone is assessed through observation of certain anatomical reference points, e.g., the scarf sign or lateral rotation of the head, or through gross estimation of a flexion curve, e.g., flexion of the trunk. In carrying out these maneuvers, the examiner must carefully control the force applied to the infant and be sensitive to any indications of resultant discomfort, representing the angulation or flexion limits.

The flapping maneuver estimates the inhibitory functions of antagonist muscle groups by assessing the amplitude of movement resulting from rapid shaking of a distal segment. This maneuver, which is useful in determining asymmetry between extremities, can be effective as well in achieving relaxation prior to the evaluation of active tone.

ACTIVE TONE

Active tone is represented in the infant's response potential to maneuvers other than muscle stretching, which explores only the passive tone. Any stimulus that activates posture and motor activity must be included in the description of active tone. In contrast to passive tone, active tone cannot be considered a singular entity. Because any definitive description would not be possible, we shall limit our discussion to a review of certain fundamentals essential to justification of the proposed examination (see Fig. 1).

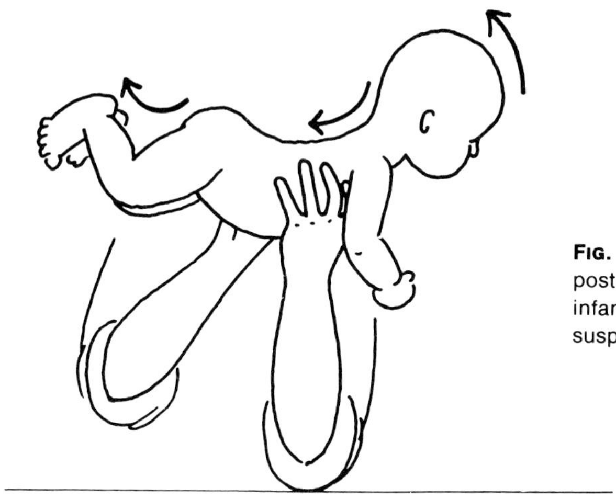

FIG. 1. Landau reflex. Total postural activity of body with infant supported in ventral suspension.

1. *Is there a resting tone*? This question does not merit debate at this point. Indeed, it is more interesting to study muscle tone abnormalities as defined by decreased or exaggerated tone. Some imprecision or confusion

might result from the use of customary terminology, e.g., hypotonia, hypertonia. Nevertheless, we shall adopt these terms and acknowledge the inherent criticisms and limitations.

2. *Is there an active tone*? The classic distinction that has been made between postural attitude–including age of appropriate head control, sitting, and standing–and locomotion–encompassing walking as well as all earlier forms of moving about, such as creeping and crawling[18,19,36]–is of some importance in underscoring the means by which active tone can be initiated. For example, if controlled by the infant, active tone is a determinant of spontaneous motor activity; if controlled by the examiner (i.e., directed motility), certain specific stimuli can vary the infant's posture and gestures. We describe those stimuli that activate the posture of the whole body, as observed in the Landau reflex (Fig. 1). Even though postural activity is included in the classic neurological examination, we refer the reader to Vojta's study of postural reflexes.[37] Vojta describes seven reflexes–Landau reflex, Vojta reflex, Peiper reflex, Collis vertical reflex, Collis horizontal reflex, response to traction test, and axillary suspension–defining the CNS postural activity as "the ability to adapt to changes of the body's position in space." Vojta describes a series of stereotyped responses that change with age, beginning with birth and culminating in the infant's ability to walk. As these changes are dynamic in nature, the motor responses provide important indications of the infant's postural and gestural organization. These dynamic responses have inspired the research of A. Grenier on certain aspects of the active tone in the newborn and infant.[14-16]

Chapter 2

Preliminary Aspects of the Neuromotor Examination

EXAMINATION OF THE SKULL–CHANGES IN HEAD CIRCUMFERENCE

Fontanelles and Sutures

Throughout the 1st year of life, the first step of a neurological examination consists of observation, palpation, and measurement of the skull. The posterior fontanelle is the first to close and usually is not palpable after 6 weeks of age. The size of the anterior fontanelle is variable, as is the age at which it closes, ranging from 10 to 20 months. Palpation of the sutures may demonstrate separation or overriding, the significance of which is dependent on the infant's age at the time of the examination.

Shape of the Skull

An elongated, narrow head, the result of sagittal suture synostosis, may lead us to suspect a craniostenosis. Coronal suture synostosis will result in a large head and flat forehead. Hydrocephaly is suspected when the anterior half of the head appears enlarged because of a prominent, bulging forehead. A large head with a prominent occiput might indicate a Dandy–Walker malformation.

Measurement of Head Circumference

Defined clinically as the maximum fronto-occipital perimeter, expressed in centimeters, this is a simple and reproducible measurement. Head circumference has been shown to correlate with head volume as measured by more sophisticated radiological examinations. The results of

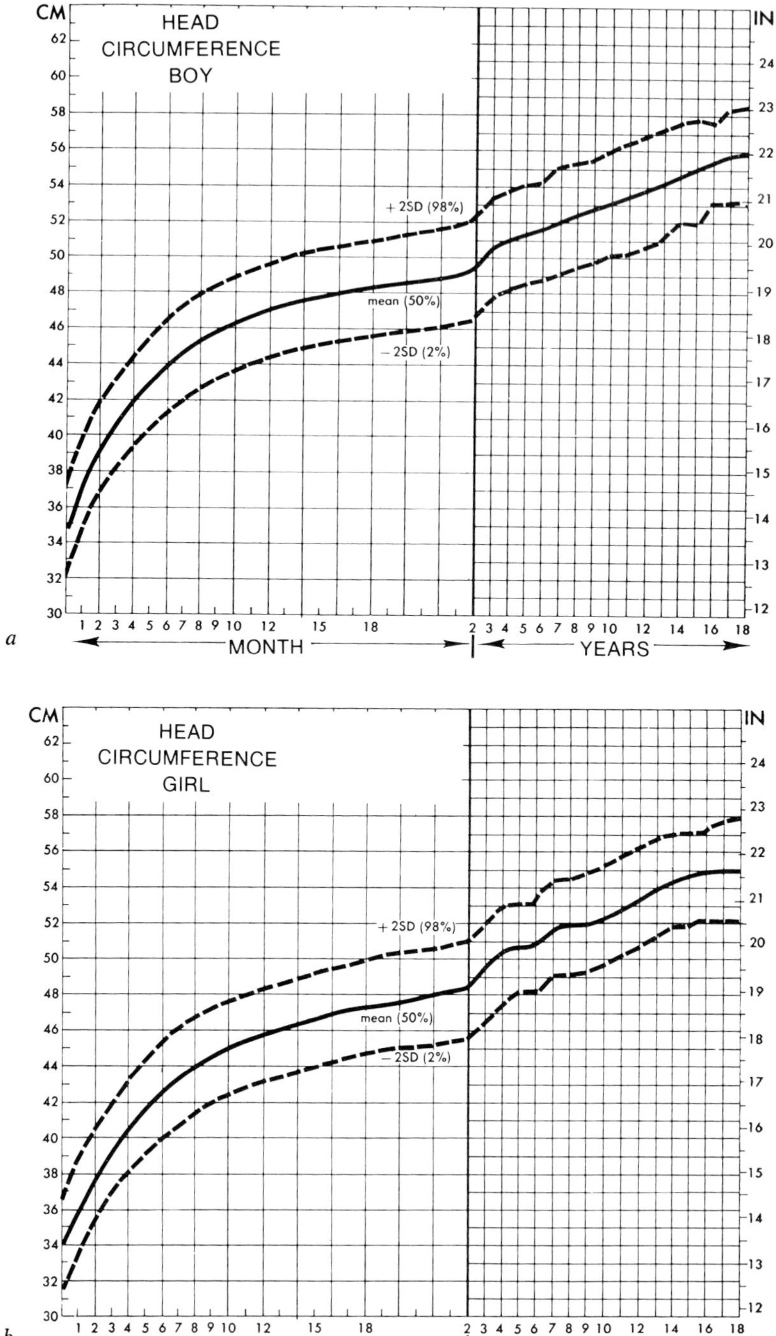

FIG. 2. Head circumference charts. a. Males. b. Females. (Nelhaus, G.: Composite international and interracial graphs. *Pediatrics* 41:106, 1968, with permission).

this measurement are to be recorded on the head circumference curve[25] (sec Fig. 2a,b).

Head Circumference Curves

Reference to head circumference curves permits identification of gross abnormalities in head circumference, defined as 2 standard deviations (SD) above (i.e., macrocephaly) or 2 SD below (i.e., microcephaly) the mean.

Transillumination

An integral part of the initial skull examination is transillumination. This may be done either with a simple pocket light fitted with a soft rubber border, or with a more sophisticated device emitting a cold light source, e.g., a chun-gun. These examinations are carried out in a dark room. Abnormal diffusion of light is apparent in the case of abnormal fluid collection. This liquid collection can be either peripheral or intracranial, as in the case of a reduced cerebral mantle. Other causes of positive transillumination include subdural effusion, cerebral atrophy, porencephaly, hydrocephaly, and hydranencephaly. The size of an acceptable halo is dependent on the intensity of the light source. When using a simple pocket light, a halo of <1 cm is considered acceptable. Cranial transillumination norms have been established for the chun-gun at specific gestational ages.[38] Reference to these norms will minimize the potential for erroneous interpretation and abusive pathologic diagnosis.

Pathologic and anatomic diagnosis can be made on the basis of history and the results of the simple examination described above. Two common diagnoses must be ruled out, however, before undertaking more complex or radiologic exploration, or both. The flat, elongated skull of the premature infant may result from prolonged molding of a soft skull positioned on a hard surface. Such molding results in a flattening of the skull, thereby creating the false impression of hydrocephaly. The familial large head–either brachycephaly or dolichocephaly–is apparent on initial examination of an otherwise normal newborn. In such instances, it would be helpful to see both parents and to investigate familial hat sizes before ordering any invasive examinations.

Auscultation

Auscultation of the scalp can demonstrate important clinical signs of an intracranial arteriovenous malformation manifested by the presence of an intense bruit. Measurement of intracranial pressure at the level of the anterior fontanelle is a simple, reliable examination used in diagnosing and monitoring intracranial hypertension.[17,39] We will not review the findings that can be obtained by lumbar puncture or ophthalmologic examination, nor will we discuss radiologic explorations, e.g., routine skull series and more complex evaluations, such as computerized axial tomography (CAT) of the skull.

EVALUATION OF STATE

Numerous studies have shown that all aspects of the neurological examination are influenced by the infant's level of alertness, i.e., the arousal state. Therefore, it is essential to define precisely the infant's state during the examination. Prechtl and Beintema[26,27] have described five states commonly used in scoring the level of alertness:

State 1 Eyes closed, regular respiration, no movements
State 2 Eyes closed, irregular respiration, no gross movement
State 3 Eyes open, no gross movements
State 4 Eyes open, gross movements, no crying
State 5 Eyes open or closed, crying

As Prechtl observed, the scoring of these states depends on the combination of heterogeneous variables. Of course, as we shall see, other combinations are possible; however, these definitions are sufficient for routine examinations. High interrater reliability has been reported. There is an optimal state for response to any given observation or maneuver. If the infant is not in a favorable state, one must either awaken or soothe the infant or postpone the examination.

COGNITIVE FUNCTIONS AND PSYCHOMOTOR TESTING

The work by Gesell[13] has opened the field of psychomotor assessment in infancy. The motor examination is based on the determination of precise milestones for the acquisition of each function (e.g., head control, sitting, crawling, standing). Establishment of mean scores and deviations from the mean have been standardized under precise conditions for each function. Therefore, deviations from the normal score may be interpreted as developmental delay. In addition to the assessment of motor development, these scales examine sensory perception, comprehension, emotional reaction, and social factors. Among the most widely used scales are the Bayley (United States)[6] and the Brunet-Lezine (France).[8] These were the only scales used in most previous longitudinal studies, as they existed prior to the development of standardized neurologic examinations.

A number of basic principles are underscored through simultaneous use of both psychomotor scales and a standardized neurologic examination:

1. Psychomotor scales indicate motor difficulties. To a great extent, infant performance on the psychomotor test is a reflection of muscle tone and motor development. Accordingly, repeated evaluations over the 1st year of life would pick up any transient motor abnormalities, as would the sequential neurologic examination.
2. It is not enough to describe motor delays as a form of developmental retardation alone. Analysis of muscle tone and the dynamic maneuvers (*vide infra*) describe both the type and the mechanism of failure in each situation, thereby introducing a richer dimension to the examination beyond simple deviation from a mean score.
3. Refined assessments of functions other than pure motor performance are also included in the psychomotor testing. There is no better standardization with regard to fine motor, emotional, and social scales.

The findings noted above suggest a complementarity between neurological and psychomotor testing. Neurological examination is carried out by the pediatrician, whereas the psychologist undertakes the psychomotor and mental testing phase of the examination. Each professional functions independently. Studies comparing the results of both methods are in progress. Whereas transient difficulties can be observed by either the pediatric neurologist or the psychologist, only the mental functions are affected in many severe mental retardation syndromes of genetic or congenital origin. In such cases, a neurological examination contributes little valuable information during the first several months. The developmental scales usually represent the first abnormal finding in the absence of an alert state.

Chapter 3

Normal Development During the First Year of Life: Identification of Anomalies and Use of the Grid

METHOD OF EXAMINATION

The neurological examination described is a simple, rapid evaluation easily administered and interpreted in general pediatric practice. The results of the examination are transcribed most effectively on a form that allows comparison with normal development at any specific time. Such a grid has been used at the Port-Royal Hospital Paris, France, for the past 5 years in monthly examinations of infants through the 1st year of life.[2,4]

The grid is presented in the logical order of the physical examination. Examination of the skull is accomplished while obtaining the history. Passive tone is analyzed as the infant lies quietly prone on the examination table. Assessment of active tone follows by testing the primary and the tendon reflexes. The examination concludes with evaluation of postural reactions. Each element of the passive tone, active tone, and reflexes is compared with normal development and is grouped according to the normal patterns for each trimester. Any abnormal result is recorded in a hatched area, thereby permitting immediate assessment of the infant's normalcy. Because each maneuver can be evaluated in a simple horizontal scan, the design permits rapid screening of the grid. This feature would prove especially useful at the end of the 1st year. It is preferable that a second person transcribe the results of the examination. This serves two purposes: 1) the examiner is able to devote full attention to the examination; and 2) objectivity is increased, in that the examiner will not be biased by the results of the previous examinations. All examinations are carried out at corrected age, thereby permitting assessment of term and preterm infants according to the same criteria.

As mentioned previously, psychomotor testing will be performed as a complement to the neuromotor examination. Therefore, our grid includes no evaluations of emotional and social variables and does not assess performance relative to object handling and fine motor activity.

PHYSICAL EXAMINATION OF THE SKULL

Head Circumference

Head circumference should be measured at each visit and recorded on the head circumference growth curve. By comparing the slope of the infant's head growth curve with that of the normal curve, it is possible to determine whether head growth approaches the normal range or whether the infant is at risk for development of either hydrocephaly or microcephaly.

Anterior Fontanelle and Sutures

Because of the variability in normal size, we indicate on the grid only whether the fontanelle is tense or depressed. The fontanelle should be palpated while the infant is in a sitting position, not crying. The normal range for suture width is a function of both the infant's age and the suture being examined. For the sagittal and parieto-occipital sutures, widths of as much as 4–5 mm may be of no significance during the first weeks of life. Separation of 4–5 mm can also be observed without significance in the portion of the metopic and coronal sutures close to the angles of the anterior fontanelle.

However, separation of 2–3 mm of the squamous suture (parietotemporal) is alarming and can be a reliable sign of intracranial hypertension. If this is suspected, the skull must be reexamined every 2–3 days in order to monitor the tension of the fontanelles, any progressive enlargement of all sutures, or a rapid increase in head size. Additional procedures should be included in the workup if there is a suspicion of hydrocephaly or intracranial hypertension. Only rarely will a single measurement be of any significance; however, repeated measurements and evaluation of the growth curve will be useful in making a diagnosis.

HISTORICAL INFORMATION COLLECTED FROM THE MOTHER

An interview with the mother is extremely important and can contribute more relevant information than is possible with a number of sophisticated procedures. Without this interview, the examination would be incomplete.

1. *Sleep patterns.* Either the mother or the nurse should be asked to make a rough estimation of the infant's usual patterns for wakefulness and sleep. Interpretation of the response is dependent on the infant's age and on the absence of nutritional problems. Three abnormal situations can be identified, each specific to a different age and developmental state:
   a. The infant sleeps for only very brief periods during the day, is agitated, and cries as soon as awake. The infant is never in a quiet, alert stage; rather, the infant appears to be in a permanent state of anxiety and discomfort. This pattern is observed most commonly during the first months of life.
   b. The infant is quiet during the day but has great difficulty falling asleep at night. Sleep is preceded by a prolonged period of drowsiness. This pattern is more often noted in the 3rd and 4th trimesters.
   c. The infant sleeps for excessively long periods—far too long for a 24-hour period. The infant is constantly drowsy. It is difficult, if not impossible, to arouse the infant completely, and the infant will remain awake for only very brief periods.

   The infant's arousal state during the tests should be noted on the form, even though this represents only an imprecise estimation of alertness. The examination should be repeated if the infant is unusually agitated, as reported by the mother, or if the behavior interferes with testing. If assessments were carried out under difficult conditions, this should be noted on the examination form.
2. *Quality of cry.* The cry should be described as normal or abnormal. Abnormal indications would include a cry that is either high-pitched, monotonous, moaning, continuous, or weak, or a cry that is accompanied by cyanosis or vasomotor instability.
3. *Sucking behavior.* Sucking/swallowing coordination should be evaluated and recorded as either normal or abnormal. It should be noted if gavage feeding is necessary or if only partial bottle feeding is possible. Frequent choking during feeding—either with or without cyanosis—should be noted on the grid.
4. *Convulsions during the preceding months.* Convulsions may be generalized or localized, febrile or nonfebrile, infantile spasms, or salaam seizures (hypsarrhythmia).

ABNORMAL OCULAR SIGNS

Hypertonia of Elevators Palpebrae Superiori

In infants with hypertonic eyelids, the upper part of the sclera and entire iris are visible; however, the globe of the eye is positioned normally. This contrasts to the setting sun sign, in which the globe is lowered abnormally into the orbit. It is essential to distinguish these two conditions, as one is not a mild form of the other. Generally, hypertonia of the elevator muscles of the upper eyelids is not an isolated finding and is observed in the context of a general hyperexcitability.

Setting Sun Sign

The setting sun sign results from a downward rotation of the ocular globes. As a result, the lower eyelids partially cover the iris and the sclera above the iris is visible. The sign may be present at all times or, in some cases, it may be elicited during the examination.

Marked Strabismus

Marked strabismus may be either convergent or divergent; unilateral or bilateral.

Sustained Nystagmus

A pendular nystagmus might be indicative of a visual deficit of either central or peripheral origin. The ocular globes do not remain directed toward an object and are constantly animated in a sustained pendular movement.

SENSORY DEVELOPMENT

Evaluation of visual and auditory function is included in the cognitive developmental assessments. However, two simple maneuvers can be carried out as part of the neurological examination during the neonatal period. Once appropriate response has been documented, the maneuvers need not be repeated.

Pursuit of Light

The infant must be in a quiet, alert state. The synergy between sucking and opening of the eyes can facilitate this observation. During the neonatal period, it is easier to evaluate pursuit of light by using a light source rather than an object. The light source can be either a small flashlight or a window emitting a moderately bright light source. The infant will direct the head toward the light source, and, if the body is turned to either side, the eyes will remain fixed on the light.

Acoustic Blink Reflex

This reflex is elicited by a hand clap at a distance of approximately 30 cm from the infant's ear. The infant will respond positively to this stimulus by blinking.

POSTURE AND SPONTANEOUS MOTOR ACTIVITY

We shall preface our discussion by reminding the reader that certain postures or movements might be present consistently, whereas others will be exhibited only occasionally, or will indicate the positions preferred by the infant. Because various prognostic importance has been attached to certain characteristics of these movements, it is essential to observe the infant carefully before assigning a diagnosis or interpreting the results.

Asymmetric Tonic Neck Reflex (Spontaneous or Postural)

This reflex is observed in an infant lying in the supine position with the head turned to one side (Fig. 3). The so-called *fencing position* is exhibited in the extension of the arm on the side toward which the face is turned; the occipital arm remains flexed. The position is reversed in the lower extremities (i.e., occipital leg extended; opposite leg flexed).

Although the asymmetric tonic neck reflex can involve both the upper and lower extremities, it is considered to be present if noted in the posture of either the arms or the legs. The reflex is observed during the first 3 months of life and can be noted intermittently from the 3rd to 6th months. It is not present in table the normal child after 6 months of age.

Abnormal Hypertonia of Neck Extensors

When the infant rests in a supine position, the neck is normally flexed, the muscles are relaxed, and there is little or no space between the cervical spine and the examination table. This is true throughout all developmental phases (Fig. 4a).

When there is a hypertonicity of the neck extensors, an infant placed in the supine position cannot lie completely flat, thereby leaving a space between the neck and the examination table (Fig. 4b). As a consequence, the infant's resting posture will assume a lateral decubitus position with a posterior extension of the head (Fig. 4c).

Note: The typically deformed head and prominent occiput of a former premature infant can complicate interpretation of this sign. In such instances, interpretation must be consistent with other signs testing the same muscle groups, e.g., repeated ventral flexion of the head; cf. below.

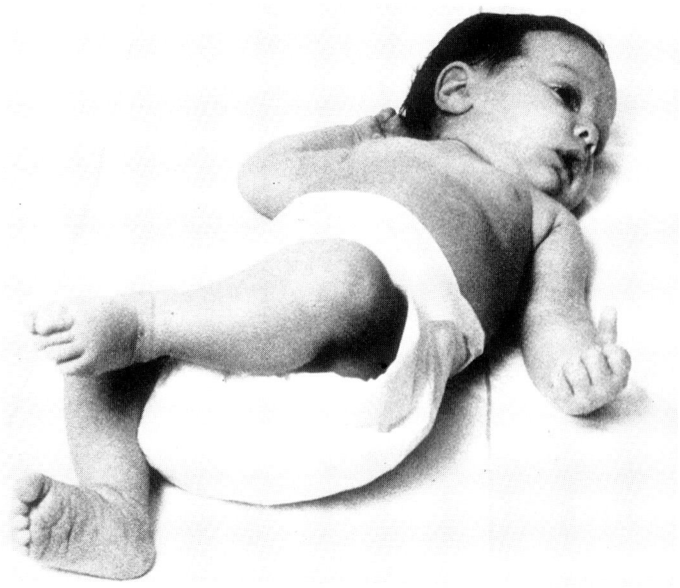

FIG. 3. Asymmetric tonic neck reflex (postural). "Fencing position" is observed in upper extremities. Extension of legs on side to which face is turned is observed less consistently.

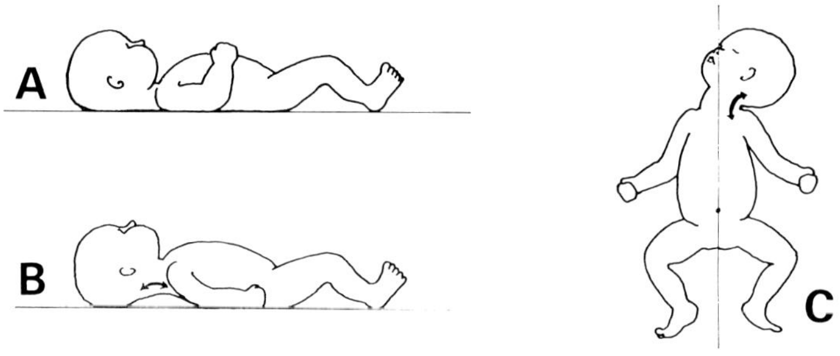

FIG. 4. Abnormal hypertonia of extensor muscles of neck. a. Normal posture: minimal free space. b. Some free space between neck and examination table. c. Resting posture in lateral rotation, with posterior extension of head in relationship to axis of trunk.

Opisthotonos

A permanent hypertonicity of the extensor muscles in the spine maintains the back in an arched position. The infant cannot lie flat in the supine position and will assume a lateral decubitus position with hyperextension when resting.

Permanent Closure of the Hands

Although the newborn's hands generally remain closed, the hands open and close continuously during sleep or while resting quietly. The hands are open most of the time after 2 months of age. Special note should be made if the thumb is adducted and flexed across the palm in the clenched fist (Fig. 5).

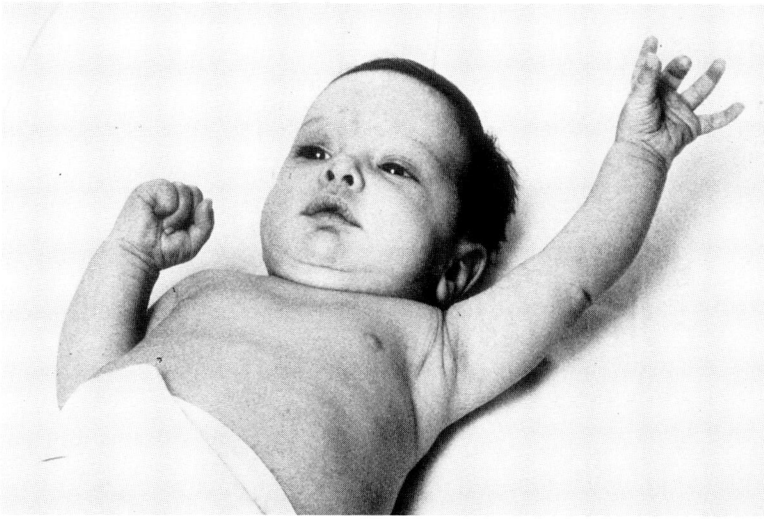

FIG. 5. Spontaneous opening and closing of hands in 2-month-old infant.

Asymmetry of Posture of Limbs

In order to determine the symmetry in the posture of the upper extremities, the head must be aligned carefully with the axis of the trunk. A permanent asymmetry in the posture would indicate asymmetry in the passive tone. This abnormality would be confirmed by specific maneuvers described later in this examination.

Facial Paralysis

Paralysis is most apparent when the infant is crying. The affected side remains flaccid or masklike, and the mouth is drawn toward the opposite side. The eye of the affected side remains partially open, whereas the eyelids close on the normal half of the face.

Spontaneous Motor Activity

Normal Movements

The infant is observed while lying supine on the examination table. The frequency and intensity of spontaneous movement are noted; however, as the examiner's observations represent no more than a gross estimate of motor activity, only significant deviations from normal are recorded. A low level of spontaneous motor activity is characterized by slow, infrequent movements and low intensity. Excessive spontaneous motor activity is expressed in frequent, rapid movements with a very high level of intensity. Normal motility is represented by a mean range in the frequency, intensity, and speed of movements.

Abnormal Movements

These can be either transient or permanent. Continuous tremors (high frequency, low amplitude) are not uncommon in term infants during the first few days of life. The tremors, which are increased by hunger and crying, are most obvious in the extremities and may be significant if persistent or present when the infant is at rest.

Bursts of Clonic Movements (Low Frequency, High Amplitude)

Bursts of clonic movements are associated with the Moro reflex or with the spontaneous motor activity of infants during the first hours of life. If the movements are noted frequently during the examination, they could be of some signficance. Other examples of abnormal motor behavior include incessant chewing movements, frequent jerking, and abnormal positioning of the arms, characterized by an extension of the elbows and pronation of the wrists.

Labile Stiffening (Dyskinetic Movements of the Limbs)

Labile stiffening can be observed during examination of the limbs. Although subject to possible criticism, the term "labile" provides an appropriate description of this finding in both active and passive movements. Stiffening may vary in intensity and duration (i.e., 10–20 seconds). The involved muscle groups may change as well. Lower extremities, including the foot, are typically hyperextended. In the upper extremities, pronation of the forearm is commonly observed. These dyskinetic movements can impede assessment of passive tone, particularly in the dorsiflexion of the foot. If pronation is present, the application of slow and rapid movements used in testing dorsiflexion must be carried out between bursts of labile stiffening.

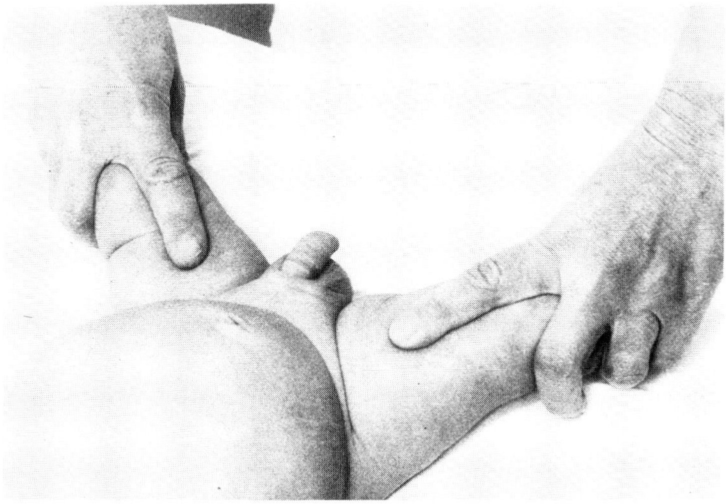

FIG. 6. Evaluation of adductors angle. Visualization of angle is simplified by placing index finger on femoral diaphysis.

PASSIVE TONE

Evaluation of passive tone is determined by the extensibility and amplitude of flapping in different segments of the extremities.

The infant's level of alertness is an important consideration in these evaluations. It is recognized, however, that optimal levels (i.e., states 3 and 4) will not be present during each examination. A less than ideal situation is acceptable, nevertheless, as the examination is proposed for use in routine office visits. Findings should be disregarded only if the infant seems to be particularly drowsy or extremely agitated. In testing extensibility, the examiner must be careful to exert no more than a moderate force. Maneuvers are stopped when the infant shows any sign of discomfort.

We have adhered to classic descriptions of the examination, the goal being to evaluate neurological function rather than to examine the joint. Asymmetry, i.e., hemisyndrome or segmental asymmetry, may be noticed during the examination.

Passive Tone of the Extremities

Adductors Angle

With the infant lying on the back, the legs are extended and gently pulled as far apart as possible. The angle formed by the legs at this point is called the adductors angle. Asymmetry between the right and left leg should be noted (Fig. 6).

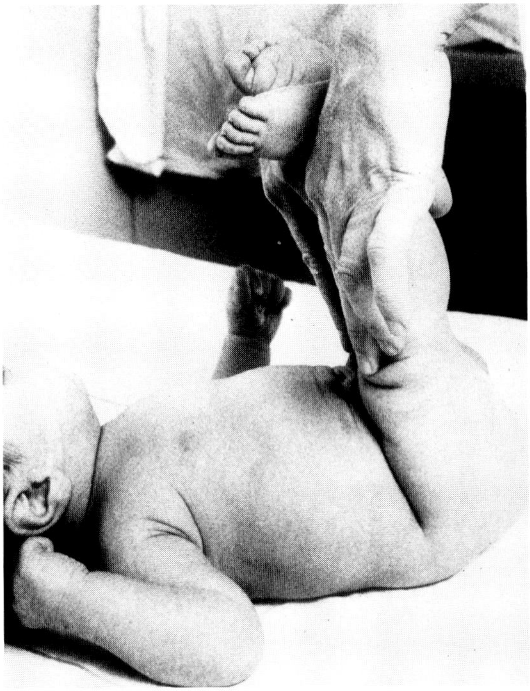

A

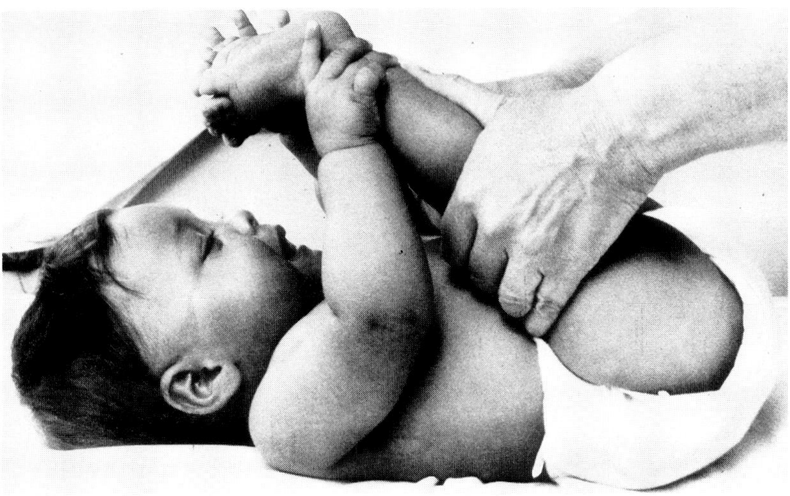

B

FIG. 7. Evaluation of heel-to-ear angle. a. 100° angle in 2-month-old infant. b. 150° angle in 9-month-old infant.

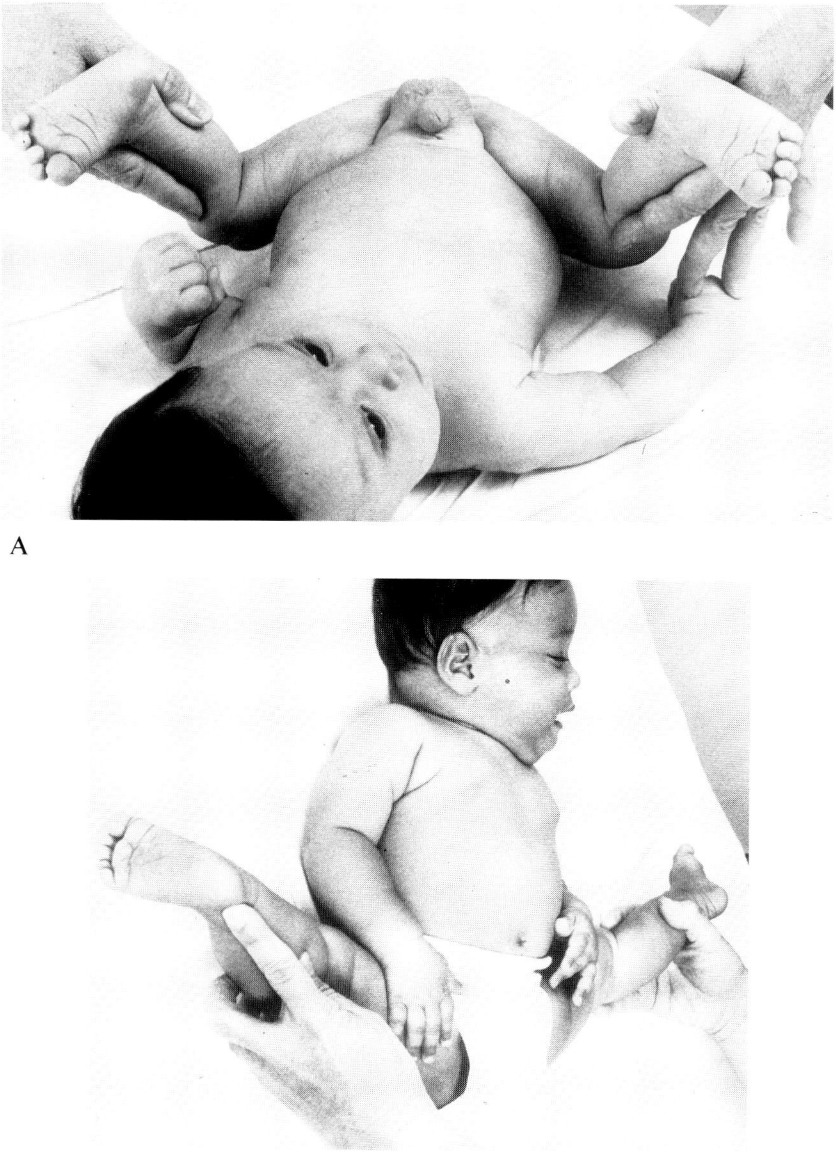

A

B

FIG. 8. Evaluation of popliteal angle. a. A 100° angle in a 2-month-old infant. b. A 160° angle in a 9-month-old infant.

Heel to Ear

With the infant lying on the back, the legs are held together and pressed as far as possible toward the ear. The pelvis must not be lifted from the table. The angle is represented in the arc extending from the infant's heels to the table. Increased resistance on one side is an indication of asymmetry, but it might be difficult to apply equal pressure to both sides.

Note: If the flexor tone is very high, complete extension of the popliteal angle might be difficult or impossible to accomplish. In this event, the angle is not that formed by the thigh and the table; rather, it is created by an imaginary line between the heel and the pelvis at the intersection with the table (Fig. 7a,b).

Hyperflexion of the Hips

If the hips are fixed in a hyperflexed posture, it will be painful or even impossible to extend the lower limbs. Such hyperflexion is considered an abnormal sign if persistent beyond the first weeks of life.

Popliteal Angle

The thighs are flexed laterally at the hip along both sides of the abdomen. While holding the infant in this position, the examiner presses the lower leg as far as possible toward the thigh. The popliteal angle, which is formed by the leg and the thigh, is estimated in both legs simultaneously. In contrast to the maneuvers described above, it is easier to apply equal pressure to both sides when examining the popliteal angle; therefore, estimation of asymmetry is more objective. Significant asymmetry is indicated by a difference of 10–20° between the right and left angles.

Note: All the preceding maneuvers may be influenced by the fetal position *in utero*. The delivery records should be reviewed if these maneuvers demonstrate extreme hyperextension of the lower extremities persistent over the first few months of life. A breech delivery or breech presentation, even after external or spontaneous rotation, may be significant (Fig. 8a,b).

Dorsiflexion Angle of the Foot

The examiner holds the infant's leg straight and flexes the foot toward the leg. This is accomplished by applying pressure with the thumb to the sole of the foot. The dorsiflexion angle is formed by the dorsum of the foot and the anterior aspect of the leg. This two-phase maneuver is carried out on each side independently. First, a slow, moderate pressure is applied to measure the smallest dorsiflexion angle, called the slow angle. This is followed by a quick, sudden flexion to determine the "rapid" angle. Normally, both angles are equal. A difference between the rapid and slow angles of more than 10° indicates an abnormally exaggerated stretch reflex.

Response to stretch. Phasic contraction, and tonic contraction: A rapid dorsiflexion movement can elicit two types of response. These can be distinguished clinically or by electromyography. The term phasic contraction is applied to a brief contraction immediately followed by relaxation. Tonic contractions are those in which a sustained resistance to the rapid movement is followed by progressive relaxation, thereby allowing a return to the slow angle.

Note: Gestational age is significant in the expression of this angle during the neonatal period and the first few months of life. Among premature infants, an angle of less than 60° would be unusual during the first year of life. This angle is measured with the knee extended in order to evaluate the whole triceps. Only the soleus muscle is tested with the knee in flexion, as the gastrocnemius muscles are excluded by flexion of the knee (Fig. 9).

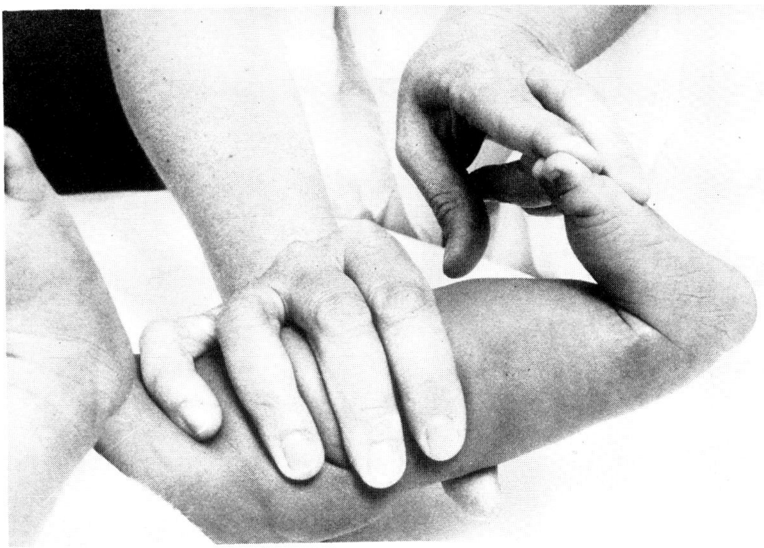

FIG. 9. Evaluation of dorsiflexion angle of foot. Flexion of foot with leg held in extension. 50° angle in 2-month-old infant.

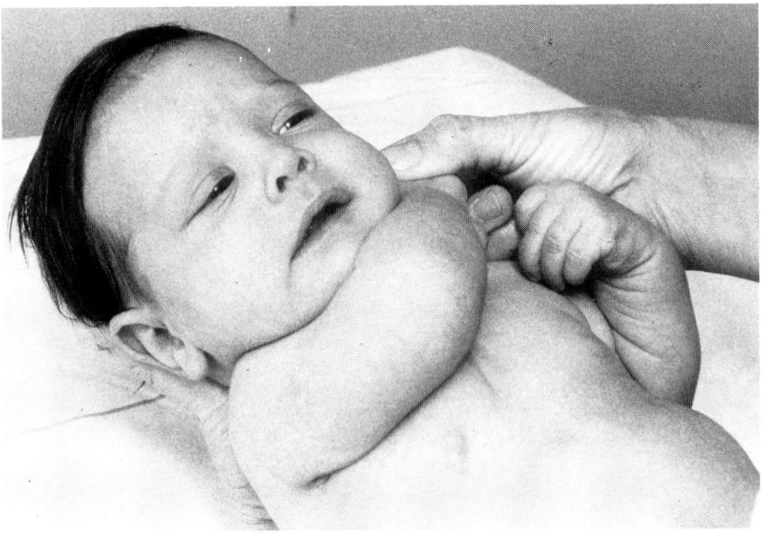

FIG. 10. Scarf sign. Infant is supported in semireclining position. Elbow reaches midline in 2-month-old infant.

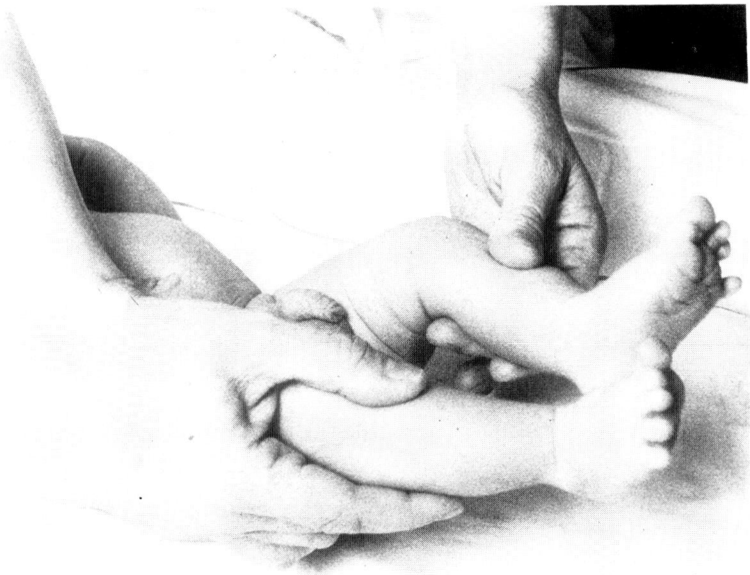

FIG. 11. Demonstration of simultaneous flapping of both feet.

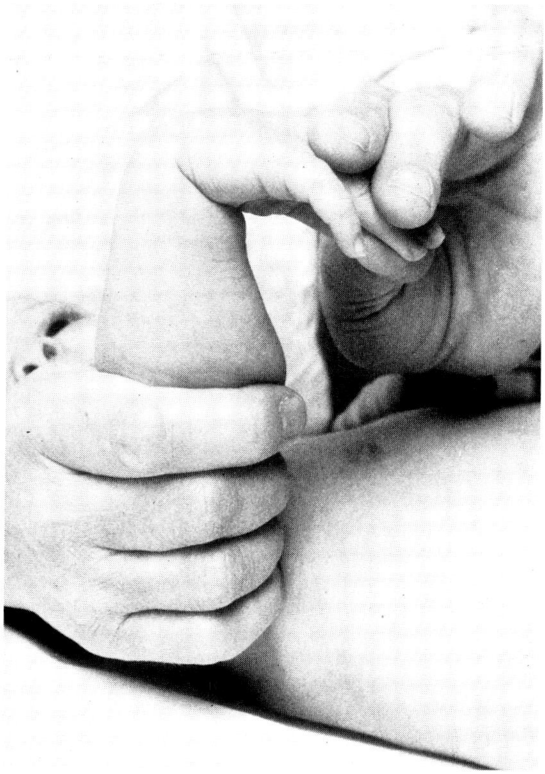

FIG. 12. Flexion of hands over forearm. Evaluation of square window.

Scarf Sign

The infant is held in a semireclining position supported by the examiner's palm. At the same time, the examiner takes the infant's hand and pulls the arm as far as possible across the chest toward the opposite shoulder. Three positions are possible in describing the position of the elbow in relationship to the umbilicus:

1. The elbow does not reach midline.
2. The elbow passes across the midline.
3. The movement is exaggerated, i.e., the arm encircles the neck like a scarf, indicating very little resistance in the shoulder muscles (Fig. 10).

Note: The scarf sign may be limited if the infant is obese or extremely irritable during the examination. If either of these conditions is present, this should be noted on the grid.

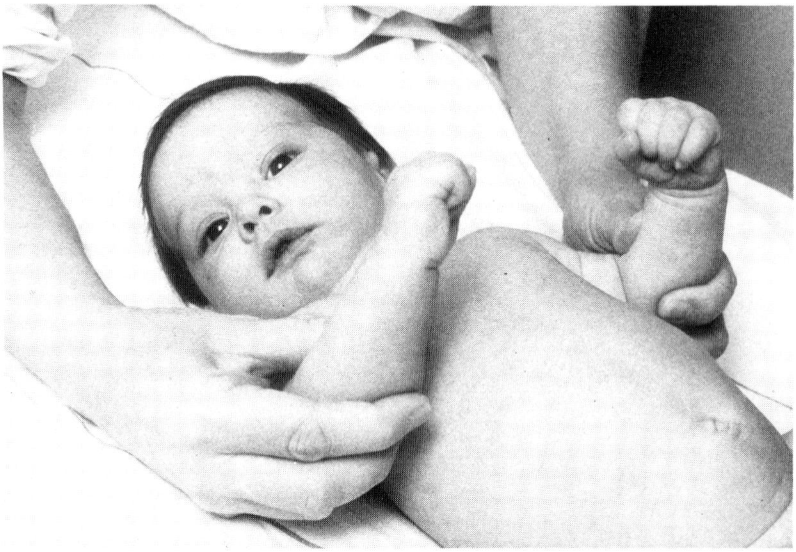

FIG. 13. Simultaneous evaluation of flapping in both hands.

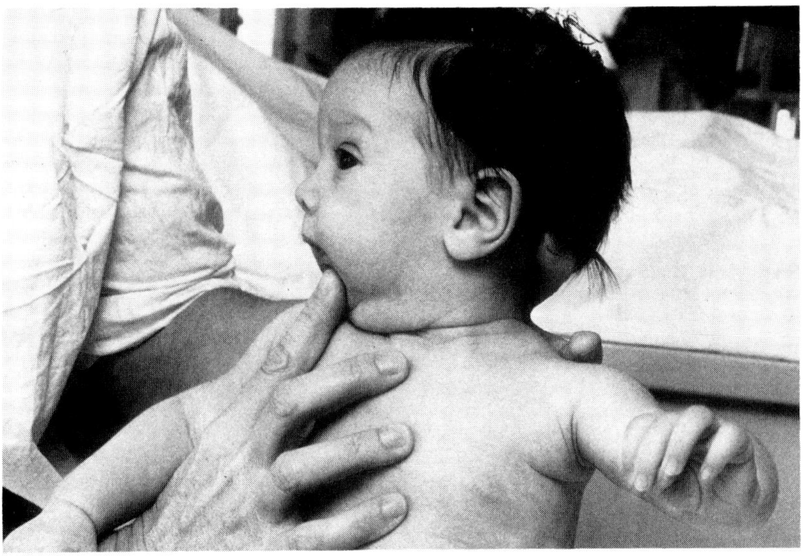

FIG. 14. Lateral rotation of head.

Flapping of the Foot

Amplitude of movement is assessed by flapping both feet simultaneously at the ankle. The examiner should note any differences between the movement in the right and left foot (Fig. 11).

Square Window

The hand is flexed as far as possible over the forearm to determine the minimum angle between the palm and the underside of the forearm. In this maneuver, we are interested in asymmetrical findings rather than amplitude of the angle (Fig. 12).

Flapping of the Hands

Both hands are flapped simultaneously at the wrist. Any significant asymmetry in the amplitude of the movement is noted (Fig. 13).

Lateral Rotation of the Head

The resistance of the contralateral muscles is evaluated by turning the head toward each shoulder. Any significant asymmetry is recorded; however, the amplitude of movement is not interpreted, as it is not important in the absence of asymmetry (Fig. 14).

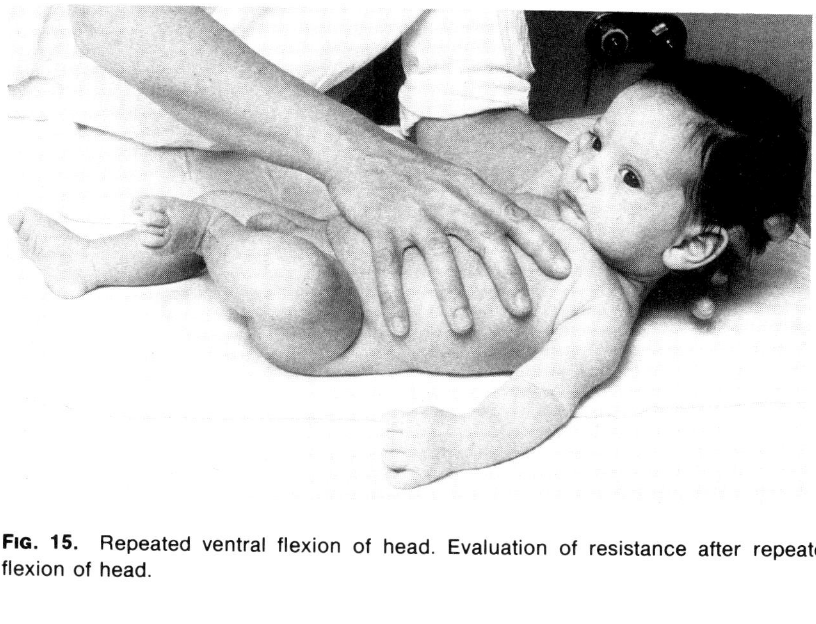

FIG. 15. Repeated ventral flexion of head. Evaluation of resistance after repeated flexion of head.

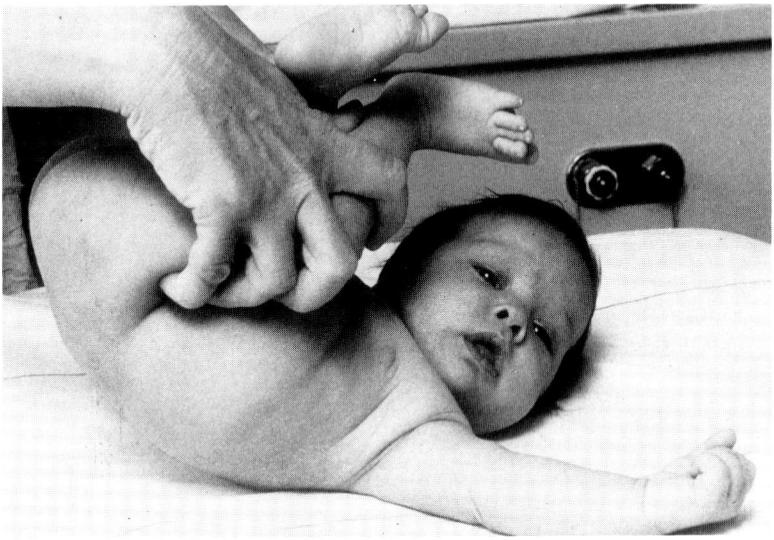

FIG. 16. Ventral flexion of trunk in 2-month-old infant.

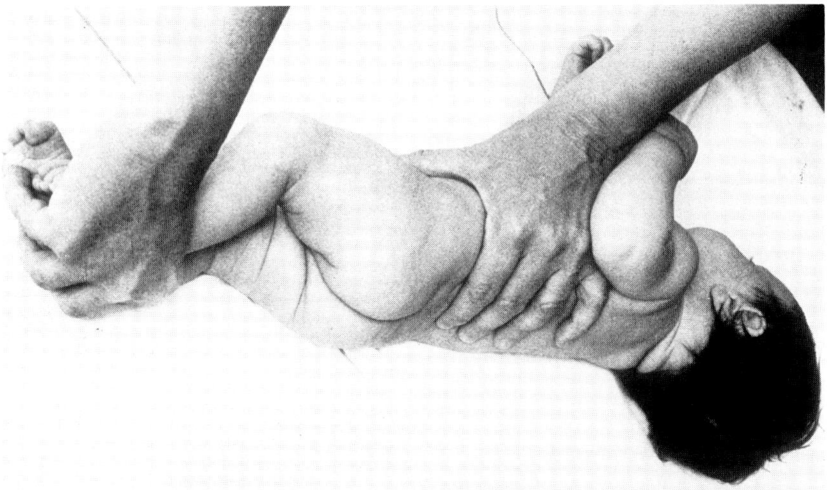

FIG. 17. Absence of incurvation of trunk in dorsal extension maneuver. One hand supports lumbar spine.

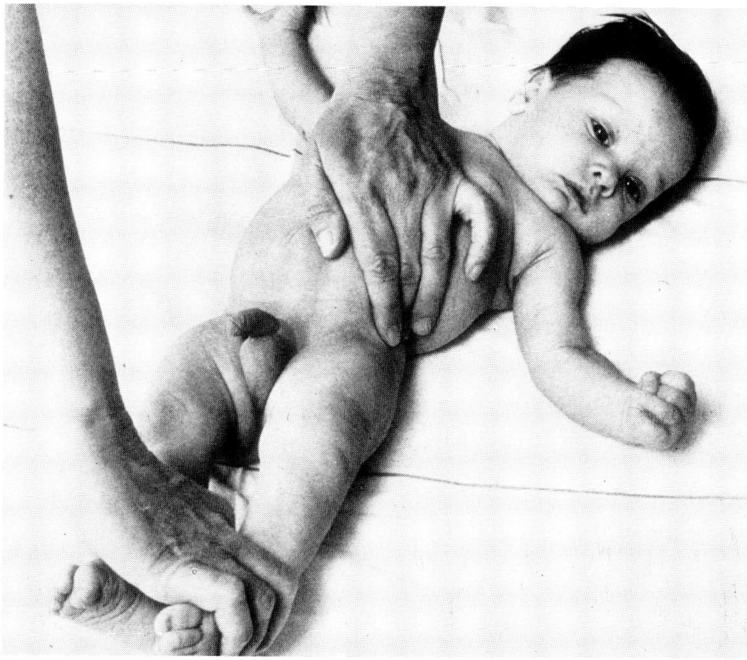

FIG. 18. Lateral flexion of trunk. One hand holds flank in position.

Passive Tone of the Spinal Axis

Repeated Ventral Flexion of the Head

Repeated flexion of the neck normally causes no changes in the resistance of antagonist muscles. Hypertonicity is indicated by increased resistance. Maximal levels are reached in most cases after four to five flexions. The head may remain fixed in hyperextension (Fig. 15).

Ventral Flexion of the Trunk

The legs and hips are pushed toward the head in order to achieve a maximum incurvation of the trunk. Some passive flexion of the trunk is normal; however, this flexion is usually limited and may be impeded further by the volume of the abdomen. If the movement is exaggerated, the knees will touch the chin without difficulty; however, flexion may be impossible. If so, the trunk remains rigid and is lifted without flexion (Fig. 16).

Extension of the Trunk (Fig. 17)

With the infant in lateral decubitus, the examiner maintains the lumbar spine and pulls both legs backward. Extension is normally very limited, if present at all. In an exaggerated response, the dorsal curve is less pronounced than the flexion curve. The absence of any extension curvature is not pathological and is considered normal at all ages.

Note: It is difficult to quantitate ventral flexion; especially so in that ventral flexion increases with age. During the third and fourth trimesters, it is not abnormal for the knees to touch the chin without difficulty. Accordingly, it is more useful to compare the relative values of the extension and flexion curves, rather than to evaluate each curve independently:

Increased flexion and extension curves are consistent with general hypotonia of the trunk.

An increased extension curve without flexion may indicate hypertonia of the spinal extensors.

Lateral Flexion of the Trunk (Fig. 18)

The infant is placed in a supine position. While holding one flank in place, the examiner pulls both legs as far as possible in that direction; thereby producing an incurvation of the trunk. This maneuver is repeated on the opposite side. Movement reflects the tonicity of the contralateral muscles and is normally very limited. Either pronounced incurvation or asymmetry would be an important finding (Fig. 18).

EVALUATION OF THE ACTIVE TONE

A signficant part of the examination grid is used for assessment of active tone. This aspect of the neuromotor examination deals with the coordinated movement of muscle groups, rather than the previously described evaluation of simple segmental responses. Evaluation of active tone is not a duplication of the passive assessments; instead, one examination complements the other.

We will refer to the neck muscles in describing the technique used to study active segmental reaction. In this example, coordinated reaction of the neck muscles is stimulated by the examiner's movement of the trunk. The appropriate speed of the movement must be acquired by experience: too brisk a motion may result in passive mobilization of the head; if the movement is too slow, the lack of active response may be interpreted incorrectly as abnormal.

When the examination is carried out appropriately, abnormal response at any age is alarming. Because of the subjectivity inherent in this evaluation, the examiner's experience is of great importance. Accordingly, conclusions should be made on the basis of repeated assessment. Integrity of motor function and the transient nature of any segmental anomaly will be confirmed by normal response to the lateral abduction reaction, as described later. If initial maneuvers reveal normal segmental response, further examinations will not be necessary.

Straightening with Neck Flexors (Pull to Sit)

The infant is grasped by the shoulders and pulled into a sitting posture. Movement from the supine position should be neither too brisk nor too slow. This maneuver elicits reaction of the neck flexors, as observed in the position of the head. Active contractions of neck flexors bring the head forward before the trunk reaches a full vertical position. Flexor and extensor tone are normally balanced in the term infant, resulting in a momentary alignment of the head and trunk prior to a forward drop of the head onto the chest. The following are considered abnormal responses to this maneuver:

It is difficult to obtain, maintain, or repeat forward flexion of the head.

The head remains passive when aligned with the axis of the trunk and falls forward immediately when brought into the full vertical position (i.e., passive forward movement).

Permanent hypertonicity of the neck extensors counters the effects of gravity, thereby preventing the head from falling forward at the end of the maneuver. In this instance, it is not possible to bring about a forward mobilization of the head, usually the easiest abnormal pattern to notice (Figs. 19a,b).

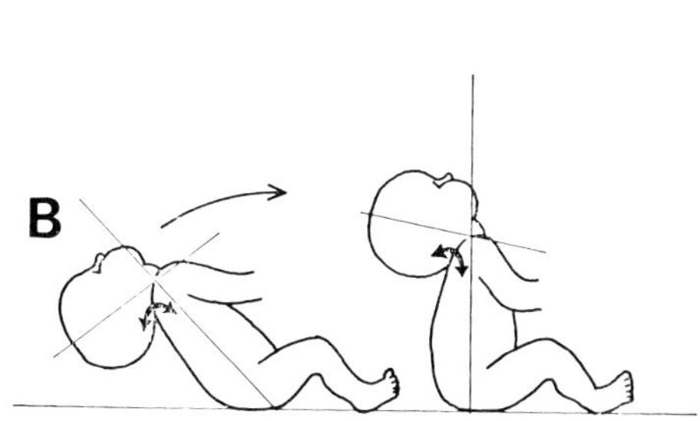

FIG. 19. Pull-to-sitting maneuver. Evaluation of neck flexor muscles: a. Normal response in term infant. b. Abnormal response attributable to imbalance of neck extensor tone. Head does not fall forward.

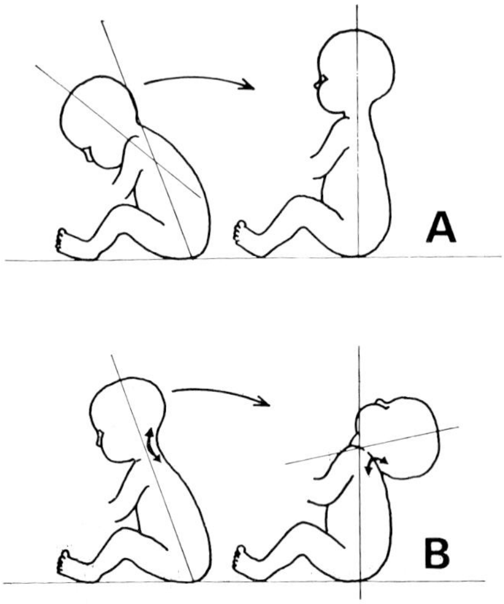

FIG. 20. Evaluation of contraction of neck extensors. Reverse pull-to-sitting maneuver: a. Normal response, head initially tilted forward. b. Abnormal response attributable to imbalance of neck extensor (increased extensor tone). At start of maneuver, head does not fall forward.

Evaluation of Neck Extensors

The maneuver begins with the infant in a sitting position, the head dropped forward onto the chest. The infant is grasped by the shoulders and moved backward. Movement must be neither too brisk nor too slow. Mobilization of the trunk should elicit contraction of the neck extensors resulting in an active lifting of the head. This reaction should be noted carefully by the examiner (Fig. 20a).

In the normal infant, an alternate contraction of the neck extensors and flexors is elicited by a gentle rocking motion at the vertical axis with the trunk. This is described as symmetrical inhibition and is normal in the full-term infant during the first days of life. The following are considered abnormal responses:

Head movement is difficult to elicit, cannot be obtained repeatedly, or is described as brisk and unbalanced.

The head falls forward over the chest at the onset of the maneuver, passes passively through the vertical axis, and succumbs immediately to the effects of gravity.

Permanent hypertonicity of neck extensors prevents the head from falling forward at the beginning of the maneuver. Movement of the trunk cause the head to drop backward immediately. The reaction is described as "too good" (Fig. 20b).

A gentle rocking of the infant at the vertical axis of the trunk will not produce a symmetrical inhibition.

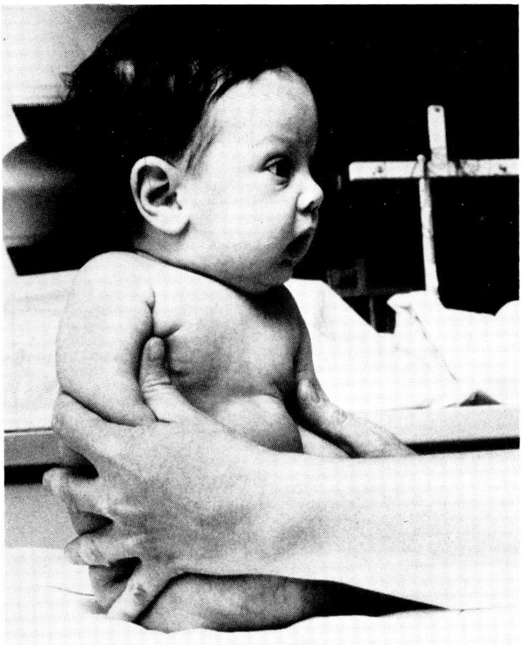

FIG. 21. Excellent head control in sitting position in 2-month-old infant.

It is difficult to examine flexors and extensors independently; however, both hypertonia and the predominance of extensor muscles may be indicated by two aspects of the previous examination (i.e., head control appears to be "too good"; the head will not drop forward). An abnormal posture, opisthotonos, is noted frequently in association with hypertonicity of the extensors.

If the extensor muscles appear predominant yet the head falls forward easily, the imbalance between the two muscle groups should be ascribed to a weakness of the flexor muscles. An ample scarf sign also may be associated with this imbalance (Fig. 20b).

Head Control

During the first several months of life, an infant placed in a sitting position cannot align the head with the axis of the trunk for more than a few seconds. The head wavers to the side or drops forward. Head control improves with age and between the second and fourth month the infant should be able to maintain head alignment for 15 seconds or more (Fig. 21).

Head control may be impossible, the result of either permanent hypertonicity of neck extensors or significant hypotonia of the neck flexors. Lack of control, in such instances, results from the absence of integrated function in both muscle groups.

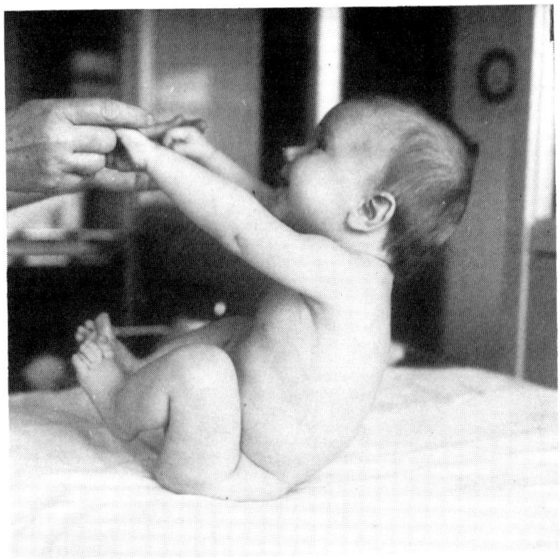

Fig. 22. Pull-to-sitting position. Five-month-old infant pulling on examiner's index fingers to achieve sitting position.

Pull-to-Sitting Position

While lying on the back, the infant is encouraged to grasp onto the examiner's thumbs. Normally, the infant will attempt to pull himself or herself into a sitting position. The examiner follows the infant's movement but provides no special assistance in attempts to achieve this posture (Fig. 22).

Note: The infant's voluntary attempt to achieve a sitting position differs considerably from the grasp and traction responses, which represent a generalized tonic flexion of all flexor muscles in the arm and forearm.

Sitting Alone, Supported by Arms

The infant is placed in a sitting position with hips adducted at approximately 90° and lower extremities in extension. The body is inclined slightly forward, leaning on the arms. It should be possible for the infant to maintain this position for several seconds (Figs. 23a,b). Two types of abnormal positions can be observed:

1. The infant may fall forward between the legs; the trunk remains completely hypotonic and no active attempt to maintain vertical position is noticed.
2. The infant might fall backward because of insufficient tone in the anterior muscle groups or excessive tone in the posterior muscle groups.

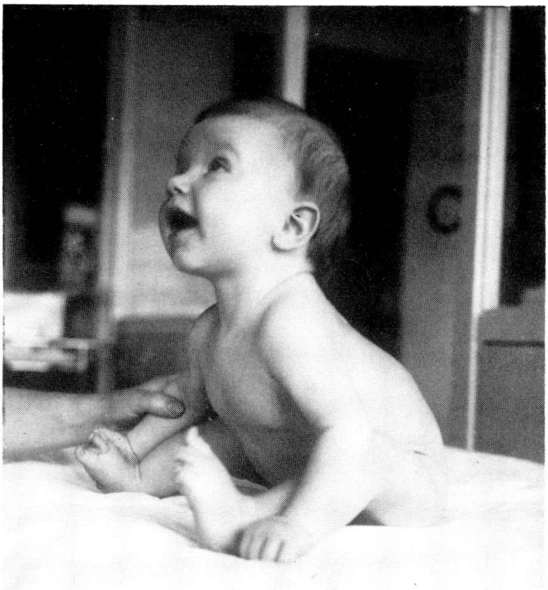

FIG. 23. Sitting alone momentarily. a. Five-month-old infant sitting alone for several seconds, using arms for support. b. Note large support base provided by abduction and extension of lower extremities. Position shown is appropriate for 5-month-old.

a

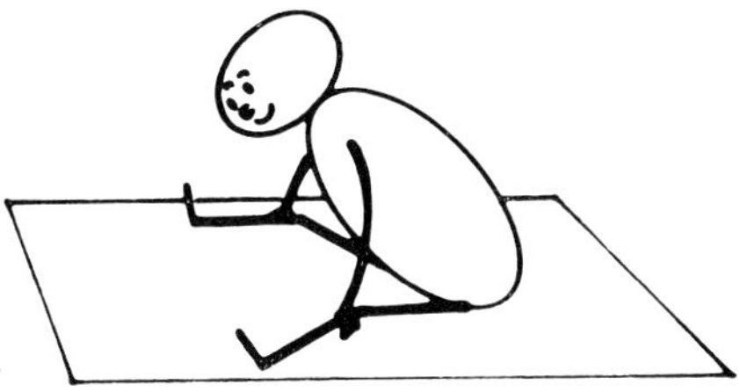

b

FIG. 24. Inability to sit alone. Sitting position is impossible. Knees are high and close together; infant falls backward.

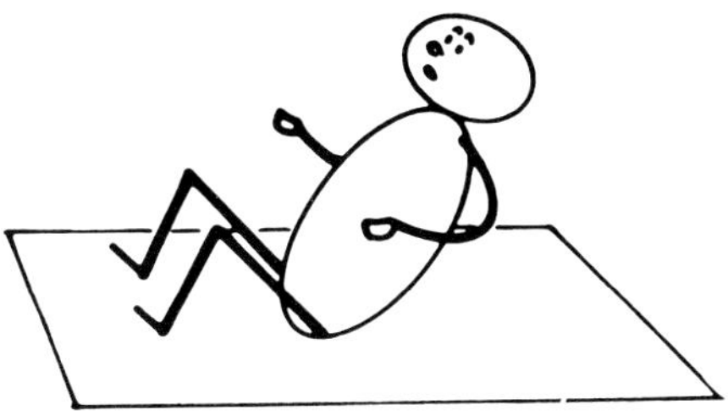

It can be difficult or impossible to place the infant in a sitting position because of decreased extensibility and abnormally strong flexor tone in the lower extremities. The knees may be too high because of a decreased popliteal angle, or the knees may be too close together as the result of a decreased adductors angle (Fig. 24). Such decreases in either angle prevent the triangulation in the lower extremities necessary to ensure a good sitting posture.

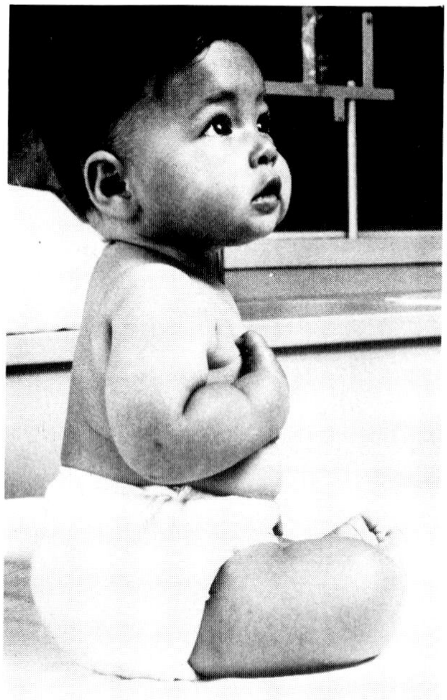

Fig. 25. Sitting alone without support. Appropriate sitting position in 9-month-old infant.

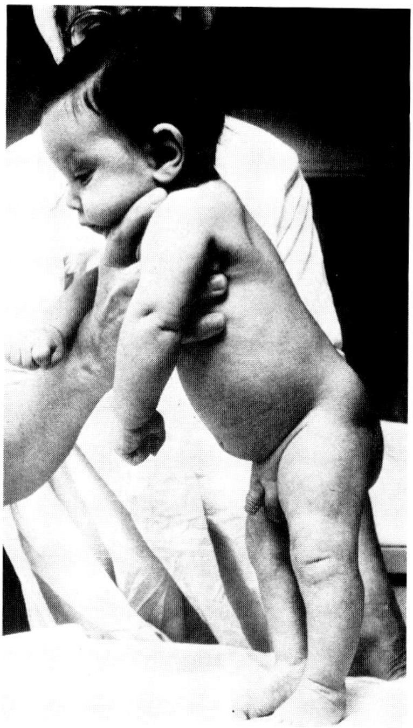

Fig. 26. Straightening with lower limbs and trunk. Two-month-old infant.

Sits Alone for 30 Seconds or More

The infant is positioned as described opposite and is able to sit for at least 30 seconds without support (Fig. 25).

Global Straightening of the Trunk

The infant is maintained in a standing position, supported by the examiner's hand around the chest. The middle finger holds the infant at the axilla and the index finger lifts the chin. By straightening the lower extremities, i.e., contracting the spinal muscles, the infant should be able to support himself or herself in this position for several seconds without additional assistance (Fig. 26).

During the first few months of life, this straightening reaction is considered present even if the knees remain semiflexed, resulting from hypertonicity of the flexor muscles. The reaction disappears over the following several months. During this time, it is impossible for the infant to stand, either by reflex reaction or by voluntary straightening (Fig. 27).

Presence of the straightening reaction represents a significant pathologic finding between 4 and 7 months of age if the infant is unable to sit. In such cases, straightening is pronounced and the legs are adducted in a scissoring position. The straightening reaction may not be apparent in the

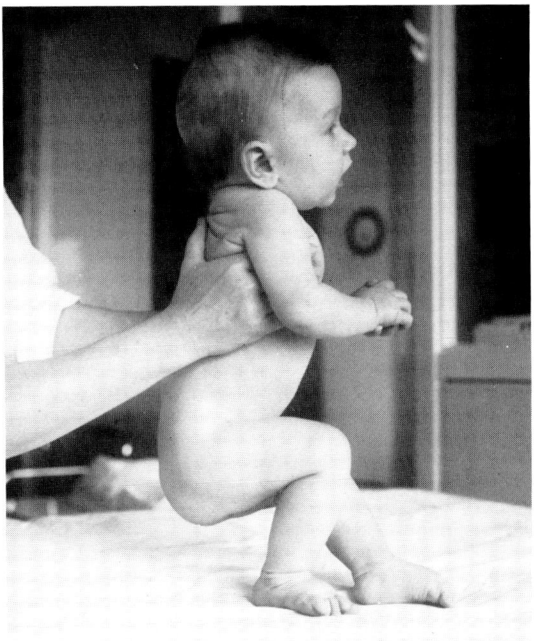

FIG. 27. Absence of straightening with lower limbs and trunk in 5-month-old infant. At this age, infant is capable of pulling to sitting position (Fig. 22) and will sit alone momentarily (Fig. 23a).

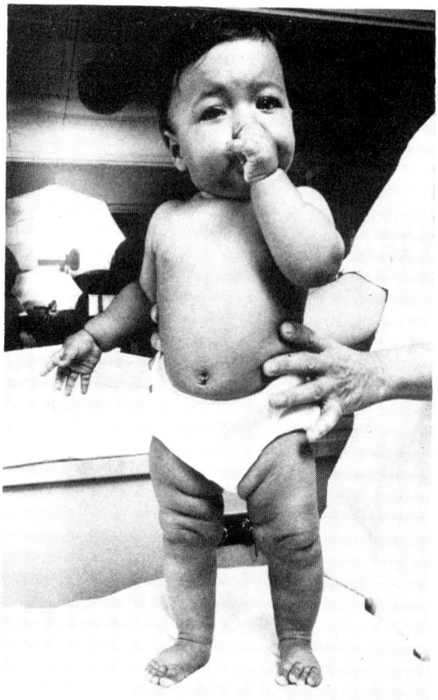

FIG. 28. Standing alone. Nine-month-old infant stands alone for extended period of time.

initial attempt, being elicited by pushing the infant's soles against the examination table. These repeated flexion/extension movements of the lower extremities may result in a very pronounced contraction of the extensor muscles.

Between 7 and 8 months, a special pattern of straightening is observed. If supported under each axilla, the infant appears unable to support his or her weight for more than a few seconds. A rapid succession of spontaneous flexion and extension movements may be observed in the lower extremities sustained as if the infant were jumping. By 8 or 9 months, the infant is capable of self-support (Fig. 28).

A marked hypertonicity of the spinal muscles may be present from birth. In this event, each attempt by the examiner to pull the infant into a sitting position will elicit an automatic reaction of global straightening with opisthotonos. This is described in the grid as trunk arching.

PRIMARY REFLEXES, DEEP TENDON REFLEXES, AND POSTURAL REACTIONS

This section describes some of the primary reflexes present during the first few months of life. While these reflexes may disappear at varying

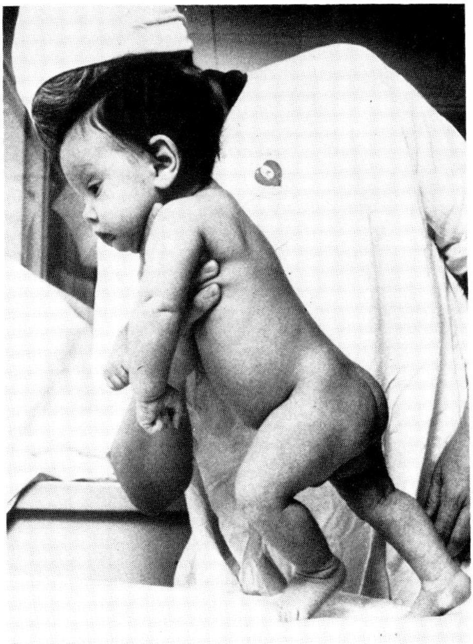

FIG. 29. Automatic walking. Two-month-old infant.

ages, persistence beyond 5 or 6 months is significant. Some deep tendon reflexes are examined routinely. In conclusion, we will describe some of the postural reactions which usually appear at a precise age.

Primary Reflexes

Automatic Walking

The infant is supported at the trunk, tilted slightly forward. Automatic walking, produced by contact of the soles of the feet with the solid surface of the examination table, is considered present when the infant takes a few steps (Fig. 29).

Automatic walking can persist beyond extinction of the straightening reaction. In this event, the infant's legs will be slightly flexed when walking.

Palmar Grasp

The examiner places an index finger in the infant's palm. This palmar stimulation produces a flexion of the fingers that decreases with age and disappears between the third and fourth months of life. The maneuver can be carried out on both sides simultaneously (Fig. 30a).

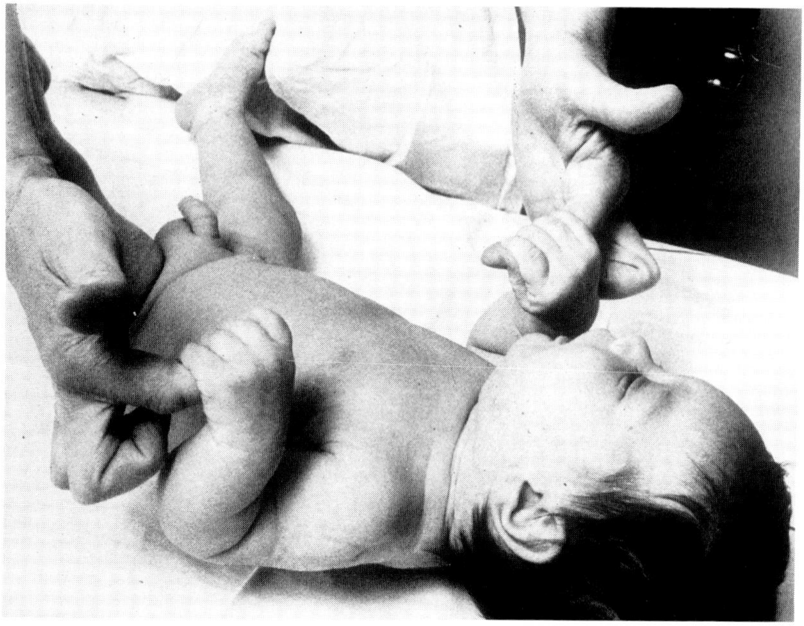

A

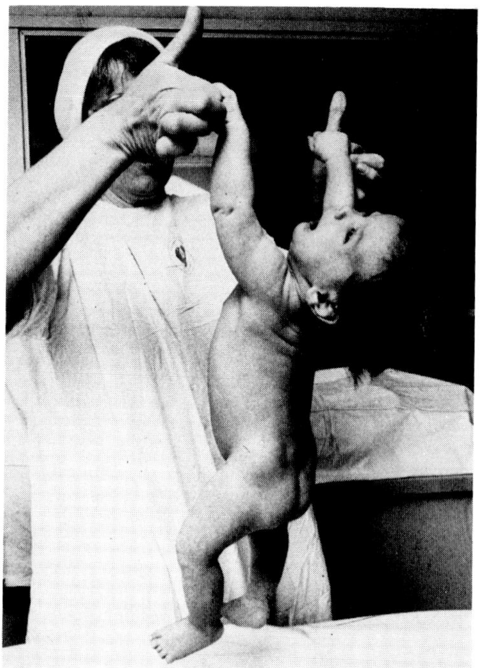

B

FIG. 30. Palmar grasp. a. Grasping reflex. b. Response to traction of flexor muscles in upper extremities. This 2-month-old infant is able to support own weight by grasping onto examiner's index finger.

Response to Traction

After eliciting the palmar grasp, the examiner pulls the infant forward–as if lifting the infant–thereby provoking a generalized contraction of flexor muscles in thc upper extremities. In this lifting reaction, the infant supports all or a portion of the weight. Tonic response of the flexor muscles is dependent on the quality of the active tone (Fig. 30b).

When general active tone is excellent, the infant's head is aligned with the axis of the trunk and the lower extremities are flexed actively for a few seconds, the infant lifting completely his or her weight in a quite spectacular way.

At the beginning of the second trimester, the two reflex reactions described above are replaced by active voluntary grasping. The infant will purposely grasp onto the examiner's index finger, pulling on this support to achieve a sitting position. Simultaneous bilateral evaluation of these maneuvers will show even mild asymmetries.

Moro Reflex

The infant is supine and lifted a few centimeters off the examination table by pulling gently on both hands. Upper extremities are in extension (Fig. 31a).

When the hands are released suddenly, the infant falls backward on the examination table and the reflex is manifest (Fig. 31b).

The reflex begins with an abduction of the arms and extension of the forearms. This is followed by adduction and flexion of the forearms. The hands open completely at the onset and the reflex concludes with the infant crying.

Normal response during the first trimester includes abduction and extension of the forearms, opening of the hands, and, finally, a cry. Adduction and flexion of the forearms may not be present. During the second trimester, the reflex may be incomplete, involving no more than an opening of the hands and a cry. Later, even this incomplete reflex will disappear. At this time, even a minimal response is considered abnormal. The examiner should be alert to the absence of the reflex during the first two trimesters, asymmetrical response, or low threshold (i.e., elicitation of the reflex by even slight stimulation). Low threshold is accompanied by a burst of clonic contractions.

Evoked Asymmetric Tonic Neck Reflex

With the infant supine, the head is rotated passively in order to change the tone of the extremities. The arm is extended on the side toward which the head is turned. The opposite arm remains in a more

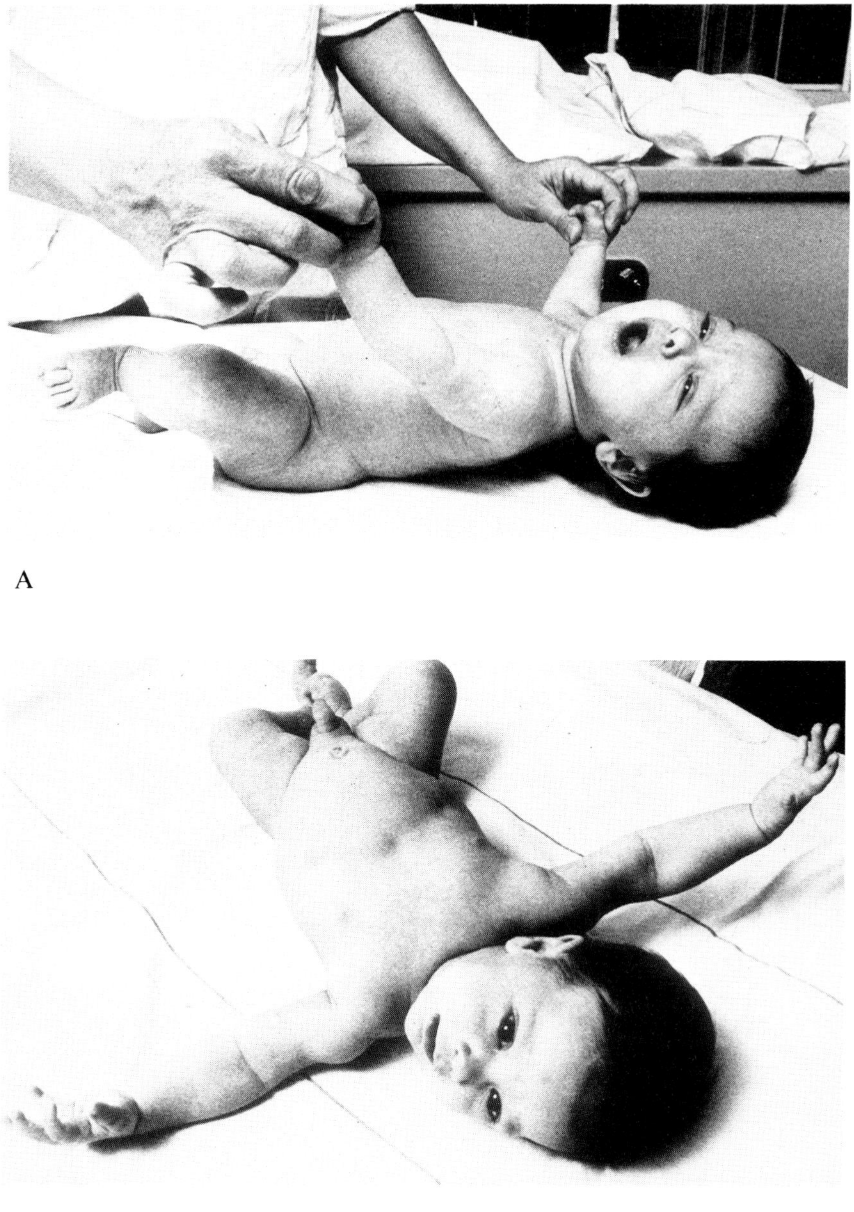

A

B

FIG. 31. Moro reflex. a. Moro reflex triggered by pulling on both hands, thereby creating space between neck and examination table. b. First phase of Moro reflex, with abduction and extension of arms. Note flexion of lower limbs; both soles turned inward.

flexed position. Only partial response may be noted in the lower extremities, which usually assume a flexion and extension pattern opposite to that seen in the upper extremities. A more detailed description of this reflex is presented on page 49. Pathologic response, never present in an otherwise normal infant, is rapid, constant, consistent, and unaffected by spontaneous motor activity.

Deep Tendon Reflexes

Biceps Reflex

With the infant lying on the back, the elbow is held in a semiflexed position. The examiner places his or her index finger on the biceps tendon. While maintaining the forearm in semiflexion, the examiner taps the index finger with a reflex hammer or with the index or third finger of the opposite hand. This tapping provokes contraction of the biceps, i.e., flexion of the forearm. Response may be absent, exaggerated, clonic, or diffused.

Knee Jerk

The infant is placed supine on the examination table and the knee is held in a semiflexed position. The reflex is elicited by tapping the patellar tendon with a reflex hammer, or with the index or third finger. Normally, sharp tap is followed by contraction of the muscle. The reflex can be absent, exaggerated, clonic, or diffused.

Ankle Clonus

The maneuver should be carried out subsequent to relaxation of the leg muscles, with the infant resting quietly on the back. A brisk but gentle dorsiflexion of the ankle is achieved with the hip and knee flexed. Ankle clonus is manifest in a rhythmic series of alternating contractions and partial relaxations of the foot at the ankle. A few rapidly fading contractions are normal in the newborn; however, a clonus persisting beyond 10 contractions is considered abnormal.

Vestibular and Visual Postural Reactions

We shall not debate the issue of whether the primary stimulus is vestibular or visual; however, it is apparent that the lateral propping reaction and parachute reaction are hallmarks of normal development. Both are of great interest clinically.

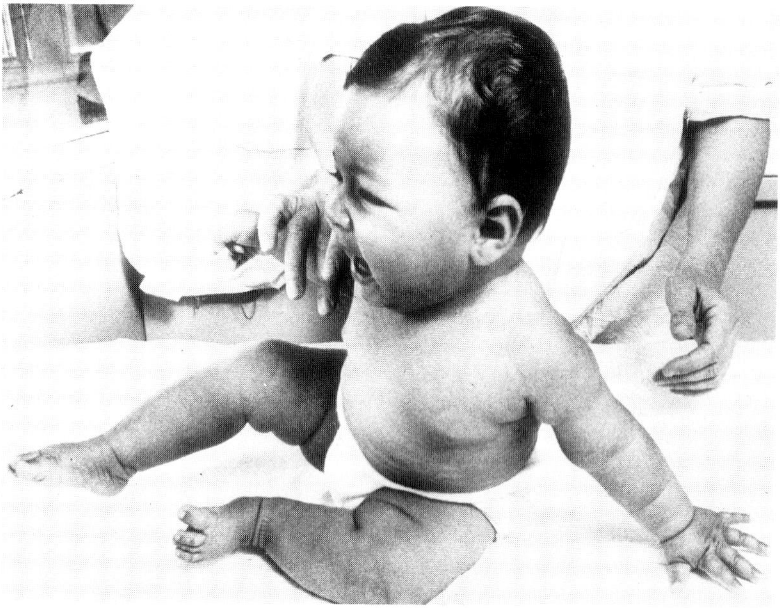

FIG. 32. Lateral propping reaction. Nine-month-old infant, sitting alone, extends one arm to prevent falling when pushed laterally by examiner.

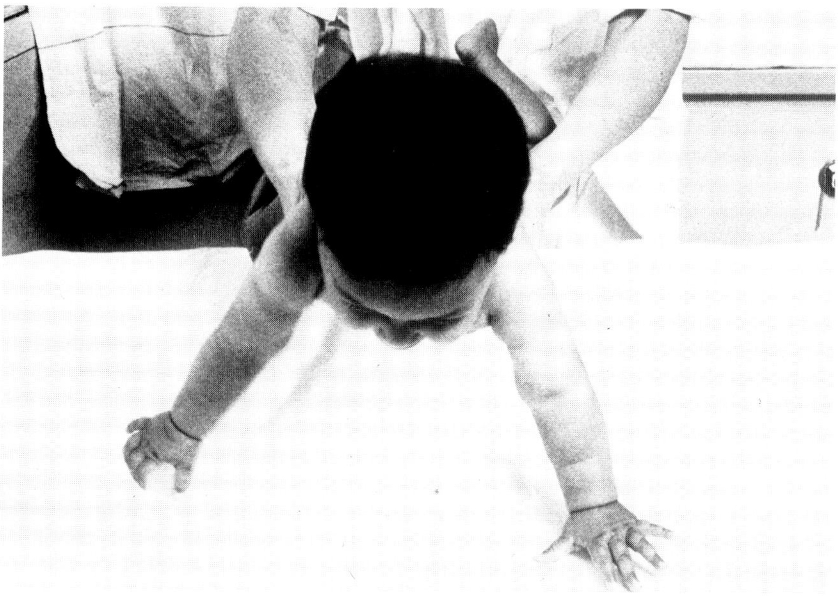

FIG. 33. Parachute maneuver. Nine-month-old infant is thrust forward abruptly toward examination table. Infant responds with protective gesture, extending arms and opening hands.

Lateral Propping Reaction

This reaction usually appears between 6 and 8 months, after the child is able to sit alone without assistance. The examiner pushes the infant to one side with a sudden shove of the shoulder. In response, the infant should extend the appropriate arm to prevent falling. Absence of the reaction or asymmetrical response should be noted (Fig. 32).

Parachute Reaction

The infant is held in ventral suspension close to the examiner, then thrust suddenly head first toward the examination table. In a normal defensive reaction, the infant extends the arms and opens the hands to break the fall (Fig. 33). This reflex appears between 7 and 9 months; however, the reaction is delayed in infants with motor difficulty of CNS origin. Absent or asymmetrical response should be recorded.

Asymmetrical findings in the two maneuvers described above are important in the diagnosis of spastic hemiplegia (Fig. 33).

CRITIQUE AND USE OF THE GRID

Each aspect of the examination can be criticized on the basis of technique and significance. In order to justify the use of particular elements of the examination, the inherent weaknesses must be understood.

Critique of Extensibility

Evolution of passive tone varies considerably among infants during the 1st year of life.[28,29] Accordingly, we must accept that normal development falls within a broad range.

It is recognized that familial hypotonicity is frequently misinterpreted. In these cases, results of the initial assessment of passive tone are inconclusive. Only after the 1st year of life is it possible to cluster the various elements of tone, thereby defining normal or pathological extensibility at any given age on the basis of all pertinent findings.

The following case histories demonstrate the difficulties encountered in interpreting these findings.

Observation 1

Elsa B. was a full-term AGA infant (4050 g). The pregnancy course was unremarkable, with the exception of a difficult forceps delivery. During the 1st week of life, several neurological abnormalities were observed.

These included an abnormal cry associated with cyanosis, hypertonia of the extensor muscles of the neck, and general hypotonia. All abnormalities, except for the hypotonia, disappeared by the end of the 1st week, and the infant appeared normal in all other respects. Head control was acquired at 4 months of age; however, abnormal passive tone was persistent at 6 months, i.e., adductors angle, 160°; heel-to-ear angle, 140°; popliteal angle, 180°. The scarf sign reached position 3 without difficulty. An exaggerated dorsal and ventral extension of the trunk was present. In questioning the mother about family medical history, she reported that one 60-year-old maternal uncle was able to put his feet behind his neck. Extensibility evolved normally within this benign general hypotonia, even though the monthly evaluation consistently revealed extensibility within the abnormal range. In this case, there is no causal relationship between the minor obstetrical complication during delivery and the observed findings. Accordingly, organic cause or perinatal etiology may be eliminated; and the prognosis, of course, would be excellent.

Observation 2

David P. was the second of twins born at 38 weeks gestation. Delivery was breech, but without difficulty. The infant weighed 2470 g at birth, was 44 cm long, and had a head circumference of 35.5 cm. Apgar scores were 8 at 1 minute and 10 at 5 minutes. At birth, there were indications of a right subdural hemorrhage. Clinical signs included a bulging asymmetrical fontanelle, widely split sutures, evidence of prior retinal hemorrhage; and permanent opisthotonos. The reflexes and state of alertness were normal, however, and the infant had a good suck. Bilateral subdural puncture was performed and 35 ml serosanguinous fluid were removed under pressure. On questioning the mother, it was learned that 2 weeks before the delivery she had fallen on her abdomen down a flight of stairs. Therefore, diagnosis of traumatic subdural hematoma was confirmed. On the days following birth, there was no reaccumulation of fluid on the right subdural space and the remainder of the infant's course was uneventful.

Nevertheless, a number of neurological abnormalities persisted. At 7 months, there were some dyskinetic movements of the lower extremities exaggerated by spontaneous motor activity. Although passive tone was normal, there was poor active tone of the trunk and opisthotonic posturing. Postural acquisition remained abnormal at 8 months. The sitting position was delayed markedly, being comparable to that of a 5-month-old infant. By 10 months, however, postural acquisitions fell within the normal range for age. Good sitting and standing positions and appropriate postural reflexes were noted.

Because of the rapid normalization between 8 and 10 months, the motor abnormalities were considered transient. Nevertheless, two aspects in

TABLE 1

Change in Patterns of Passive Tone in the Lower Extremities–Case 2: DAVID P., Ages 4–8 Months and Abrupt Return to Normal Patterns at 10 Months[a]

Adductors angle				100	100		110	130		150		
Heel to ear				100	100		110	110		140		
Popliteal angle				100	100		110	120		170		
	1	2	3	4	5	6	7	8	9	10	11	12

[a]Age in months is indicated at the bottom of each column.

the evolution of passive tone must be taken into consideration: (1) evolution of tone in the lower extremities was not smooth and regular, with tone changing abruptly between 8 and 10 months (Table 1); (2) examination of the other twin, who would serve as a control, demonstrated that this infant was normal in all respects at birth.

Over the first 8 months, extensibility in the second twin was greater, falling within the upper limits of normal for age; but, at 10 months, extensibility in both infants was identical. The "abnormal" infant had caught up suddenly with his normal twin. While the angles fell consistently within the normal range during the first 8 months of life, the patterns of evolution cannot be interpreted as smooth and normal, as

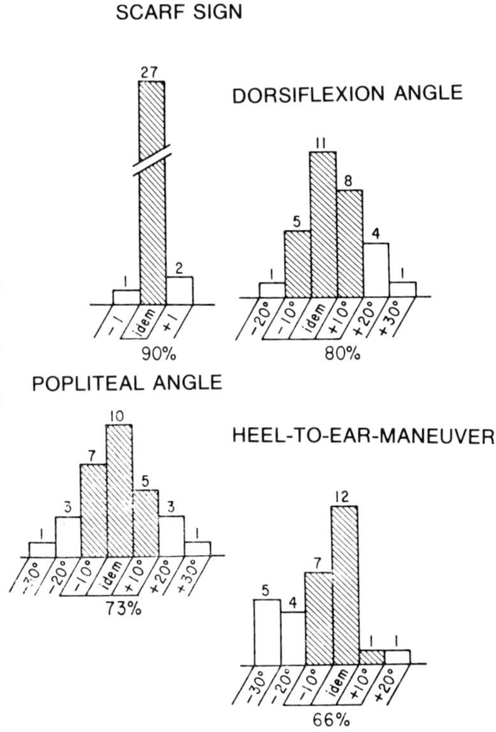

FIG. 34. Reliability in evaluation of passive tone. Results were obtained by several examiners who evaluated scarf sign, dorsiflexion angle of foot, popliteal angle, and heel-to-ear maneuver in 30 infants.

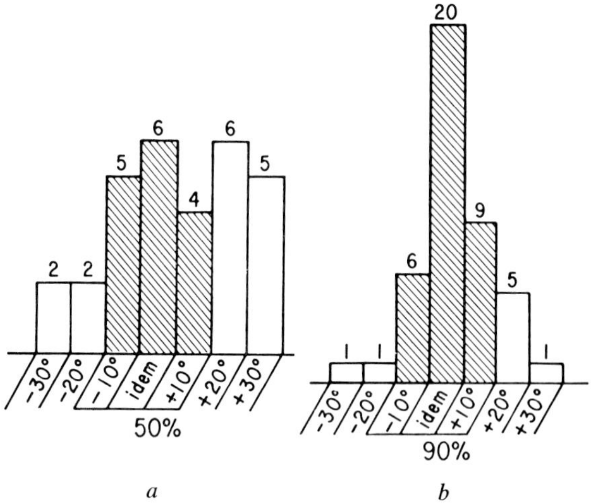

FIG. 35. Reliability in evaluation of passive tone. a. Estimation of adductors angle. Successive examination of one infant by several different examiners. b. Estimation of adductors angle when maneuver is carried out by one examiner and evaluated by several independent observers.

illustrated by the abrupt and delayed change at 10 months. It appears that the relative hypertonia normalized at the time these transient anomalies most commonly disappear. Even though no differences existed between the twins at 10 months, it would be important to follow the development of the younger twin until school age. In doing so, any subsequent developmental delays could be related to the transient motor anomalies resulting from prenatal trauma.

These two observations point out the need for correct interpretation of findings and the danger inherent in viewing raw data out of context. In case 1, conclusions based on isolated findings suggested abnormal development rather than the correct diagnosis of benign familial hypotonia. By contrast, assessments of the infant in case 2 indicated normal development, whereas patterns would have been interpreted correctly as transient anomalies related to prenatal injury.

Interobserver Reliability

Evaluation of interobserver reliability was undertaken in order to test variability between individual observers and to assess the impact of observer experience.[2]

During the first phase of the study, one infant was examined by two independent observers. Reliability proved excellent for the scarf sign and dorsiflexion angle (plus or minus 10°); acceptable for the popliteal angle;

and mediocre for the heel-to-ear maneuver and adductors angles (Figs. 34 and 35).

During the second phase, the maneuver to assess the adductors angle was carried out by one examiner; however, five independent observers concurrently estimated the angle. Results of this evaluation provided a much improved reliability (plus or minus 10°) (Fig. 35b). This example illustrates clearly that the difficulty does not lie in the visual evaluation of the angle; rather, reliability is dependent on the patience and experience of the observer. These findings also suggest that the use of measurement instruments (e.g., a compass or special device) would be less effective than cvisual estimates by a sufficiently experienced examiner. Accordingly, it is important that 1st-year evaluations of each infant be carried out by the same examiner, if possible.

SOME SPECIAL COMMENTS ON THE AXIAL TONE

Hypotonicity of the Neck Flexor Muscles

Usually, the anterior flexor muscle groups, rather than the posterior extensor muscle groups, are the first affected by anomalies in axial tone. In this instance, one observes an imbalance in favor of the extensor muscles. Major anomalies result in a significant and permanent opisthotonos. Both head control and sitting are impossible. If one attempts to produce a sitting position, the infant will rise to standing and the body will retain the pronounced incurvation. This finding is observed in association with extensive cerebral necrosis secondary to post-asphyxial damage.

Anomalies of moderate severity result in delayed head control and minor abnormalities may be detected only by an imbalance between the dorsal extension of the trunk and a relatively limited ventral flexion. This minor symptomatology will soften and disappear slowly as development progresses.

Hypertonicity of Neck Extensors and Extensors of the Trunk

A different significance is attached to hypertonicity of the extensors. Such tonal abnormalities are the best indicators of intracranial hypertension in the newborn, equivalent to stiffness of the neck in the older child and the adult. If present, the head cannot pass midline in the straightening with the neck flexor maneuver and cannot fall forward on the chest if the infant is maintained in forward flexion. The head is held back by the hypertonic neck extensors. It must be recognized that this is a very labile sign and may disappear within hours after a lumbar puncture or the use of diuretics.[3]

It is difficult to make a distinction between the two origins of axial imbalance in that the clinical examination is based on an evaluation of one antagonist muscle group in comparison with the other. Moreover, the situations may overlap, as in the case of acute fetal asphyxia in the term infant. For example, during the first few days of life, cerebral edema will result in intracranial hypertension. Permanent hyperextension of the neck will be present because of hypertonia of the extensors. Subsequently, any cellular lesion is evidenced by a weakness of the flexor muscles, thereby maintaining the relative imbalance between the two muscle groups. Straightening with neck flexors will remain poor. Backward movement of the head will appear better than forward movement; however, forward fall of the head will become possible and repeated flexion will no longer result in a progressive block. Whereas the importance of these clinical distinctions might be debatable, the increased use of electromyography may provide a more precise differentiation between the two situations. Prolonged hypotonia of the neck flexors because of cellular injury may persist concomitant to hypertonicity of the neck extensors. At the same time, hypertonia of the extensors will be present until intracranial hypertension has been resolved.

SUMMARY AND CLASSIFICATION OF FINDINGS DURING THE FIRST YEAR

Analysis and Synthesis

Although this method of neurological evaluation has not been standardized, the range for normal development and the acceptable limits are based on findings reported in the literature. As noted previously, the major difficulty in interpreting these results is attributable to the wide variations in individual tone. For this reason, it would not be appropriate to group together all the items included on the grid. Some typical neurological profiles can be identified by grouping certain of the findings, and the isolation of particular clusters of signs is a necessary step in the synthesis. At the end of the text, we provide a quarterly summary according to the age at which the signs were observed.

First Trimester

The most frequent moderate anomalies can be clustered in two groups: 1) hyperexcitability and 2) hypotonia of the upper half of the body, including poor neck flexor tone and excessive relaxation of the upper extremities. In most cases, these signs will disappear abruptly during the third month. When the infant is examined at 3 months of age, head control is present, i.e., normal for this age, and the hyperexcitability is no longer in evidence. The mother is often quite aware of these signs and may recall exactly when the symptoms disappeared. Because limited extensibility is normal at this stage, it is not possible to predict the potential for relaxation in the lower extremities. Identification of asymmetry before 3 months of age, usually indicative of spastic hemiplegia, is possible only through additional dynamic maneuvers.

In the case of extensive cerebral lesions, the early clinical signs are much more alarming and may include poor interaction, swallowing difficulties, low intensity spontaneous motor activity, general hypotonia, or permanent opisthotonos. It is apparent in these rare cases that such anomalies will not disappear during the 1st year of life.

Second and Third Trimesters

The most characteristic clustering of signs during this period includes persistent hyperexcitability, active primary reflexes, absence of change in the passive tone of the lower extremities, an imbalance between axial tone and the hypotonia of the flexor muscles of the trunk, and a relative hypertonia of the extensor muscles of the trunk. Although these anomalies might mimic spastic diplegia, the conditions can be distinguished on the basis of several findings. In true spastic diplegia, the adductors angle is very limited, with a scissoring of the legs apparent, and "tonic response to stretch" will be noted in the triceps. By contrast, a large adductors angle and phasic contractions in the triceps are generally predictive of transient anomalies. Such signs disappear spectacularly around the 8th or 9th months and the motor examination is normal at 1 year.

Subtle spastic hemiplegia of perinatal origin, which may not be diagnosed until the 5th month of life, will become more pronounced during the 6th and 7th months and disappear completely before the end of the 1st year. Table 2 outlines the most frequent symptomatic clusters and potential patterns for normalization. One might conclude that if a monthly exam is not possible, it would be most crucial to evaluate the infant during the 2nd, 7th, and 12th months, corrected age. These three examination periods yield the highest potential for identification of transient anomalies. After the first 10 months of life, it is no longer possible to distinguish those infants who became normal by that time from those who remained normal throughout the 1st year.

Other concurrent psychomotor assessments may demonstrate either normal or moderately abnormal development, or findings may prove inconclusive. In the case of transient anomalies, there is usually close agreement between the results of the neurological examinations and

TABLE 2
Most Commonly Observed Transient Neuromotor Anomolies in the 1st Year of Life

Anomalies		*Normalization*
Hyperexcitability Anomalies of axial tone (imbalance between extensor and flexor muscles of the head)	First Trimester 2 months	Head control normal at 3 months
Hyperexcitability Persistence of reflexes Absence of relaxation in passive tone of lower extremities Anomalies of axial tone The infant is unable to sit (falls backward) Persistence in straightening of lower limbs and trunk	Second and Third Trimesters Less frequently 4th trimester 7 months	Relaxation of lower limbs Normal sitting position Appearance of postural reactions at a normal or slightly delayed date
Cerebral palsy Spastic diplegia Spastic hemiplegia Quadriplegia Choreoathetoses	Anomalies persisting at the end of the 1st year 1 year	

psychomotor assessment. The neurological examination may be incapable of identifying instances of mental retardation in which there are no motor disabilities; however, complications at birth rarely result in this type of retardation. By synthesizing findings at the end of the first year, we are able to classify infants according to the following criteria:

1. Normal throughout the 1st year

2. Transient anomalies
3. Persistent anomalies

SIGNIFICANCE OF TRANSIENT MOTOR ANOMALIES

Correlation of Findings with Difficulties at School Age

It is not possible to establish a prognosis for each infant solely on the basis of the limited data generated by 1st-year neurological evaluations. At the same time, it would not be feasible to wait until the child reaches school age in order to assess the impact of neonatal intensive care, to gauge yearly progress in clinical care within such a unit, or to compare infant outcome across centers. By school age, more than one-half the infant population will have been lost to follow-up. Among those remaining, it would be necessary to group children according to socioeconomic classifications in order to assess the impact of cultural and environmental factors. Moreover, because significant changes in clinical management would evolve over a 7-year interval, the results of longitudinal follow-up studies would not be pertinent to current care practices. In order to circumvent these difficulties, researchers have focused more intensively on the relatively narrow and precise range of neuromotor development in the first 12 months of life.

We have learned to recognize certain neurological anomalies and have discovered that the physiognomy of these anomalies differs during the various developmental stages. We know that some infants may experience transient anomalies and that by the end of the 1st year it is no longer possible to distinguish such infants from those who have remained normal since birth. However, experience has shown such normalization to be deceptive in that it is attributable only to a certain developmental threshold. Cell damage of perinatal origin is very likely present in both white matter and gray substance. Given the kind of functioning that cannot, as yet, be explored, white matter deficit can be detected more rapidly than that of gray substance. Therefore the damage will be manifest again in the following years, typically in the form of behavioral difficulties, fine motor anomalies, or subnormal IQ.

Perinatal pathology would seem to represent the obvious link between transient anomalies and difficulties at school age. Moreover, this causal association confirms the organic basis of subsequent difficulties. If neurological testing were not carried out in the 1st year, the organic basis of school-age problems would be difficult to confirm, as such problems are often vague and may be attributed to various factors.

In 1972, Drillien described a cluster of transient anomalies found in a group of low birthweight (1000–1500 g) infants.[10] These anomalies were followed by normalization of motor findings at 1 year of age. Study infants were evaluated until school age and were compared with two control groups. The first group consisted of infants of the same birthweight who had not experienced motor anomalies during the first 12 months. There was a second control group of healthy term infants.[11] Six infants in whom cerebral palsy developed were excluded from the study. All others were subjected to a battery of tests between 6 and 8 years of age. A handicap score, ranging from 0 to 3, was calculated on the basis of school performance, IQ, and motor/perceptual difficulties. Roughly, those infants with a handicap score of 0–1 were well adapted in school; children with minor problems were scored at level 2; and a score of 3 was attributed to children with more significant difficulties. Control infants were matched for socioeconomic classification. The following results were reported: There were no differences in school performance between low-birthweight infants without 1st-year motor difficulties and term control infants. However, among the infants with transient anomalies during the 1st year of life, 23% had handicap scores of 3. By contrast, a handicap score of 3 was assigned to only 9% of the low-birthweight group without motor anomalies and 4% of the full-term controls (Table 3).

These data, which were generated in a large infant population, are the first to validate the correlation between first-year neuromotor signs and subsequent school performance. More recent investigations at Port Royal Hospital, Paris, France, are being undertaken among term infants who have experienced obstetrical trauma. At this point, none of the infants has reached school age; however, preliminary findings suggest that transient signs in this group are similar to those described by Drillien in the premature infant.

Although severe cerebral palsy is easily recognized and may be diagnosed as early as the first few months of life, such early diagnosis is rare even in the very small premature infant. Evaluation of transient motor

TABLE 3

Extent of Handicap as Expressed by a Total Score, Determined by a Battery of Tests Between 6 and 8 Years[a,b]

Final Handicap Score	*Neurologic Abnormalities (%)*	*No Neurologic Abnormalities (%)*	*Controls (%)*
0	31	55	68
1	33	28	16
2	13	8	12
3	23	9	4
Number of cases	100	131	111

[a]Reproduced with permission: Drillien, C.M. in: *Major Mental Handicap. Ciba Foundation Symposium*, No. 59. Elsevier, New York, 1978.

[b]Subjects included low-birthweight infants who experienced motor anomalies during the 1st year of life, low-birthweight infants with no motor anomalies during the first year of life, and a control group.

difficulties is of great importance in determining the impact of neonatal intensive care on intact survival of the CNS.

Other groups have reported similar correlations between motor difficulties during the 1st year of life and subsequent minimal brain dysfunction.[9,23] Minor lesions resulting in transient motor difficulties in low-birthweight and high-risk infants are much more common than permanent motor handicaps. Drillien reports 100 transient anomalies, but only six cases of cerebral palsy.

WHY DO SOME MOTOR ANOMALIES NORMALIZE DURING THE FIRST YEAR OF LIFE?

A number of studies have suggested that there is a dormant period between the ages of 1 and 5. It should be noted, however, that normalization at around 10 months of age involves only gross motor development. Fine motor development remains poor, and both language and behavior develop abnormally. However, it is difficult to demonstrate, quantify, or classify these findings. A more precise clinical examination would make it possible to establish a pathological link at the various developmental stages between 1 and 5 years.

The high incidence of minimal brain dysfunction among infants who experience transient 1st-year motor difficulties establishes a causal relationship and confirms the organic origin of abnormal signs at school age. Indeed, the transient motor signs represent a minor form a cerebral palsy, i.e., a minor form of leukomalacia. Leukomalacia may result from isolated lesions; however, as reported by Banker and Larroche, these are most frequently associated with concomitant cortical lesions.[5] It appears, therefore, that mild lesions of the white matter result in transient anomalies during the initial stages of development. Cortical lesions become evident later and will determine the long-term prognosis.

These clinical and anatomical hypotheses were confirmed by computed tomography in 46 children (ages 4–15) diagnosed as having minimal brain dysfunction.[7] Some atrophy of the cortex or other cerebral areas was present in 32% (15) of these infants.

Chapter 4

Additional Neuromotor Examination: Lateral Abduction Reaction of the Lower Limb Obtained by a Hemilateral Progressive Motor Reaction (Directed Motor Activity)

LATERAL ABDUCTION REACTION

We have developed an additional neuromotor assessment of the newborn and infant as a means of enhancing the methodology of the classic neuromotor examination. Specifically, this component of the examination addresses the need for a prognostic assessment of the later motor function during the first 3 months of life. The lateral abduction reaction combines a series of dynamic maneuvers (i.e., rotation, straightening, and spatial movement), which activate all aspects of active tone and are intended to provoke a series of gestures and postural changes. The examiner initiates and guides all these maneuvers and evaluates the level of organization, integration, and control evidenced by the infant. Such directed motor activity has been employed by a number of investigators who have developed structured examination procedures.[21,22,32,33,37,40]

This postural reaction elicits a series of muscular contractions in a cephalocaudal progression along one side of the body, terminating in an abduction of the hip. Whereas the response is always absent in infants with cerebral palsy, the presence of this reaction confirms normal neuromotor function and is predictive of neuromotor potential. Because anomalies in the early neurological examination may prove transient, this maneuver is especially important in those infants evidencing such initial signs.

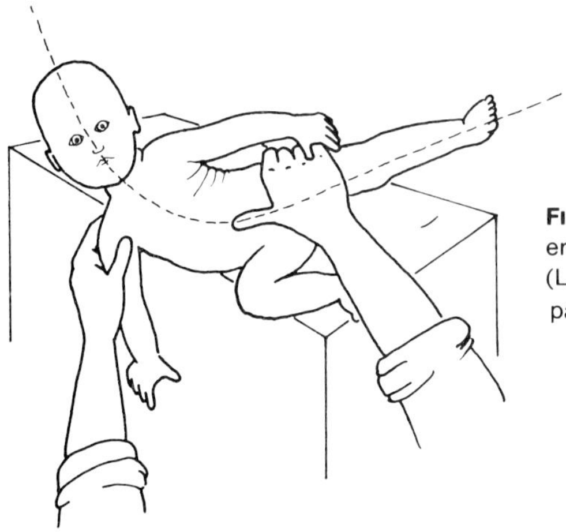

FIG. 36. Schematic drawing of lateral abduction reaction of hip. (LAR) (A. Grenier maneuver) Cf. pages 60 and 61.

CLINICAL DEMONSTRATION

The lateral abduction reaction may be present as early as the first days of life; when it is not evident, however, a series of maneuvers may be carried out to encourage the response. Such maneuvers may stimulate or actually foster development of the reaction. Indeed, we have observed that the reaction has been induced in numerous cases involving infants having no initial response.

Described below are the techniques employed in examining the reaction, as well as those to be followed in inducing the response. The examination techniques consist of the following procedures:

1. The maneuver begins with an active lateral straightening of the head by the examiner. This straightening is intended to initiate postural reactions manifest in a series of active contractions involving all of one side of the body, including the lower extremities (Fig. 36).
2. The role of the examiner is crucial in
    a. Controlling and directing the active contractions, thereby limiting these to only one-half the body.
    b. Maintaining complete extension in one of the lower extremities.

Clinical demonstration of this examination technique merits a detailed description. We shall describe successively 1) the sequence of maneuvers and responses, 2) special precautions, 3) examination technique, and 4) common errors in technique and interpretation.

SEQUENCE OF MANEUVERS AND RESPONSES

Starting Position

The infant is first tilted on the table facing the examiner, then placed in a strict lateral decubitus position without support to the head (Fig. 37). The limb placed below is held in a flexed position, thereby preventing its involvement in the expected motor reaction. The other leg is maintained in full extension (see below). In order to evaluate motor response in the lateral abduction reaction, it is essential that this starting position be maintained precisely throughout the examination.

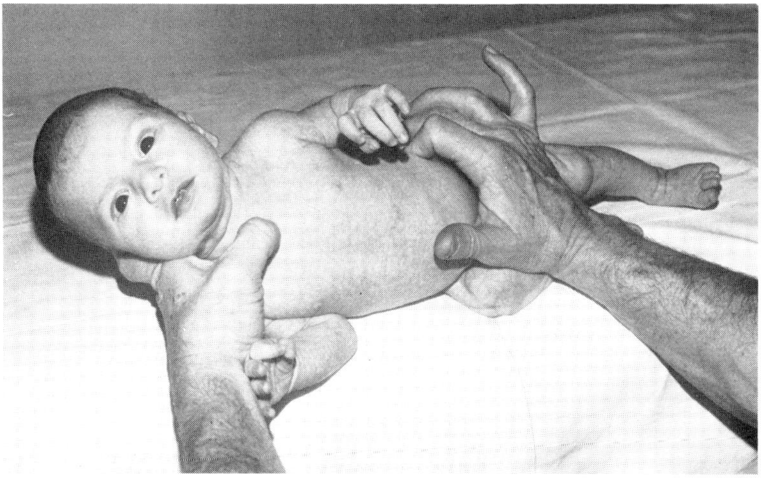

FIG. 37. Lateral abduction reaction: Starting position. Lateral abduction is not yet present. Infant remains in lateral decubitus, without support to head. Bottom leg is flexed; top leg is extended.

Activating Maneuver

Response is triggered by moving the head from side to side (Fig. 38). The actual technique used in moving the head varies according to the infant's age and will be described later.

Progressive Response

One must observe very carefully the movement of the head and the sequence of contractions as they progress through the entire body (Figs. 38 and 39). The contractions begin with the neck; produce a lateral incurvation of the trunk, extending through the pelvis, thigh, and leg; and culminate in dorsiflexion of the foot. The toes are pointed toward the examiner.

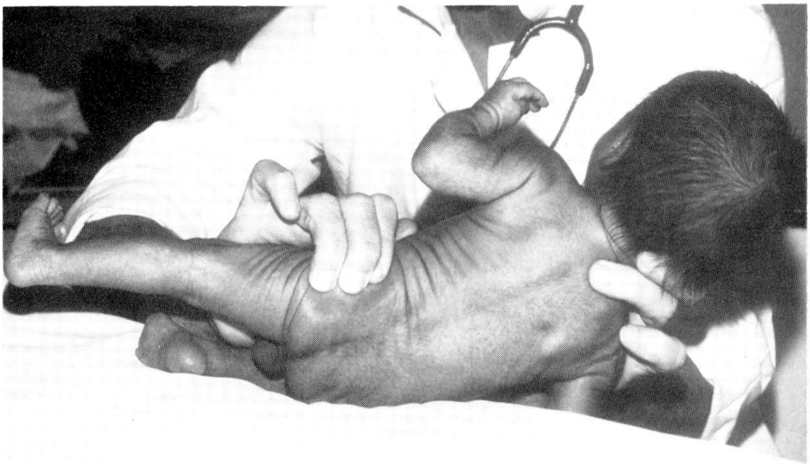

FIG. 38. Lateral abduction reaction: Start of reaction. Examiner flexes infant's head laterally several times. Abduction is not yet present.

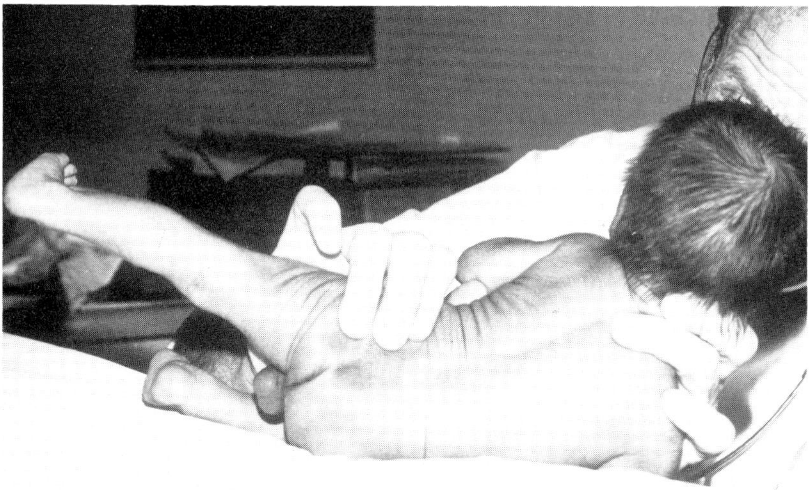

FIG. 39. Lateral abduction reaction: Reaction development. Observe lateral straightening of head; chain reaction of contractions along trunk; leg extension; and changing position of foot (dorsiflexion of foot with toes pointing toward examiner).

Culminating Abduction of the Hip

Lateral abduction of the hip may be observed only after having carefully established the position of the lower extremity. The entire extremity is lifted by contraction of the abductor muscles in the hip being examined (Figs. 40 and 41).

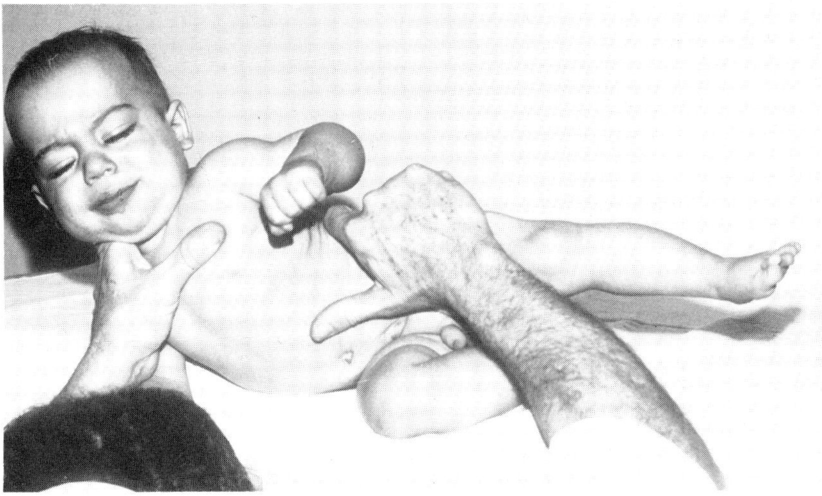

FIG. 40. Lateral abduction reaction: Culminating response in chain of contractions. Takes place along trunk. Correct position is assured; extended leg is about to lift.

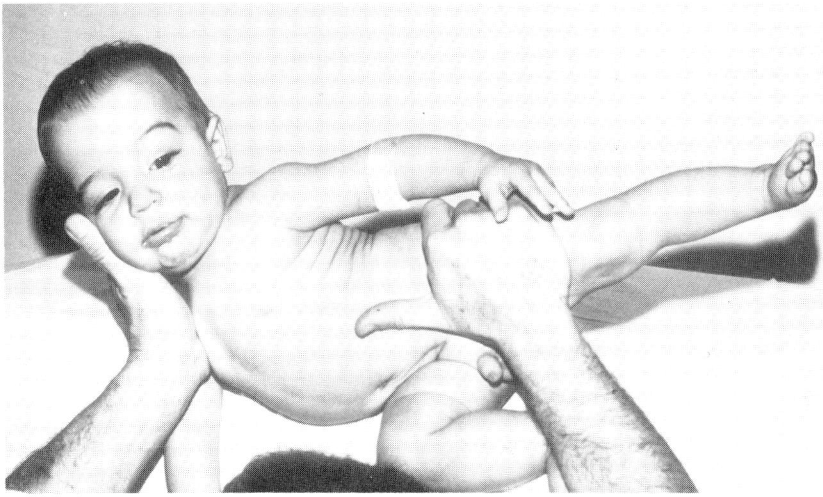

FIG. 41. Lateral abduction reaction: Culminating response, description. Leg is merely lifted in abduction, without flexion of hip and knee. Infants tolerate maneuver without crying and without fighting (hand is open, infant is relaxed).

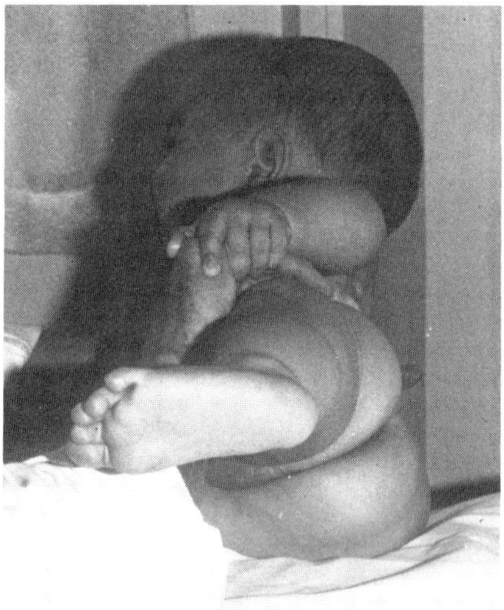

FIG. 42. Lateral abduction reaction: Alignment of axis of trunk with neck and leg. Imaginary line intersects earlobe, midline of lateral aspect of hip, knee, and external malleola.

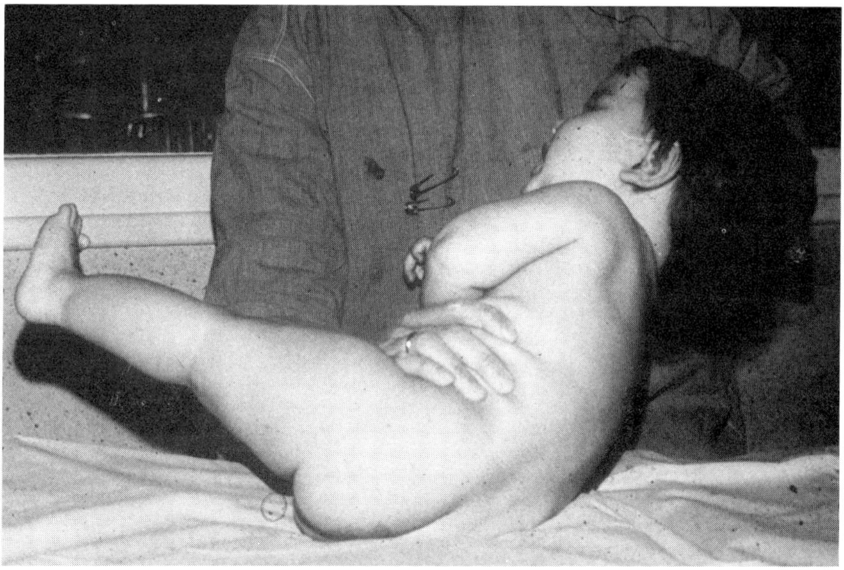

FIG. 43. Lateral abduction reaction: False abduction. Hip is flexed over pelvis, thereby invalidating reaction. Flexor muscles are activated by chain reaction, rather than by abductor muscles.

SPECIAL PRECAUTIONS

Axial Alignment

The hip must be aligned in direct extension with the pelvis (i.e., the axis of the body must be aligned with the end of the lower extremity).

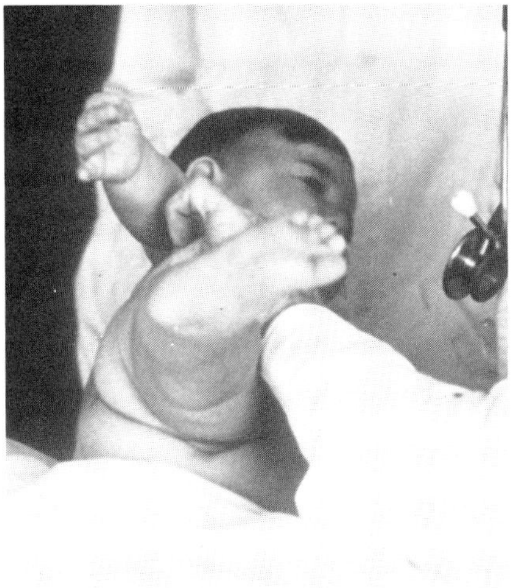

FIG. 44. Lateral abduction reaction: Falsified response. Note external rotation of foot. Toes are pointing upward, in response to flexor muscles of hip, rather than to abductor muscles.

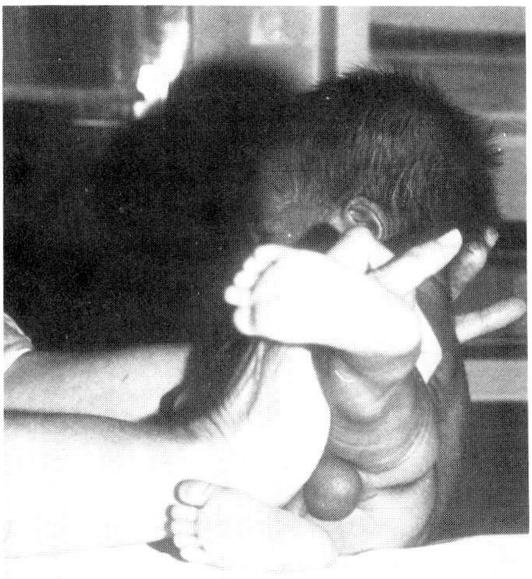

FIG. 45. Lateral abduction reaction: Correct horizontal position of foot. Toes pointed toward examiner.

This is necessary in order to assure that the mobilization of the lower extremity results solely from contraction of the abductor muscles of the hip. To ensure correct positioning during the examination, the examiner should envision a straight line intersecting with the earlobe, the external malleolus, the center of the lateral aspect of the hip, and the knee (Fig. 42). If this alignment is not exact, response to the maneuver cannot be interpreted. Even a slight flexion of the hip will result in hip elevation by the flexor rather than abductor muscles. This false abduction would constitute an incorrect interpretation of the reaction (Fig. 43).

Even greater care must be taken to assure the alignment of the trunk and the lower extremity. Correct interpretation of the reaction is not possible if there is any deviation from this alignment (e.g., flexion of the head; incurvation of the trunk; flexion of the hip or knee; external rotation or upward direction of the foot), thereby allowing flexor contraction of the hip (Figs. 44 and 45). In order to overcome these difficulties, modifications in the maneuver have been suggested for the very young infant (page 70). Because spontaneous flexion of the hip over the pelvis is present in this population, it is imperative that the examiner maintain the lower extremity in extension throughout the examination.

Repeated Lateral Flexion of the Head

The head movements triggering the reaction must be continued until the infant responds by flexion of the lower extremities. As the head is moved laterally toward the shoulder, the face is maintained in a strict forward position without rotation of the neck (Fig. 46). The actual technique used in carrying out this maneuver is dependent on the infant's age and postural abilities.

1. When the infant is capable of managing good head control, the examiner will tilt the head without actually touching it. The head is lifted spontaneously and held in this position by repeated muscle contractions. These repeated contractions maintain horizontal alignment of the eyes (Fig. 47) and result in head movement triggering the lateral abduction reaction.

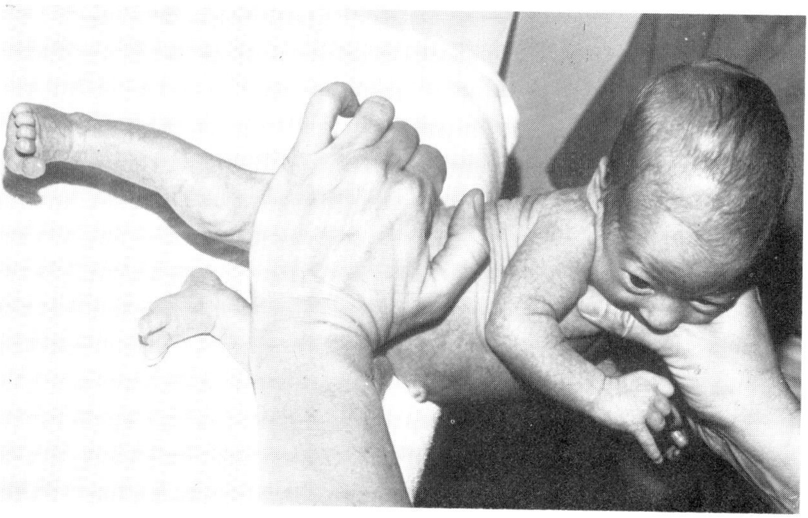

FIG. 46. Lateral abduction reaction: Lateral movements of head (rotation). Ear is inclined directly toward shoulder without rotation of neck.

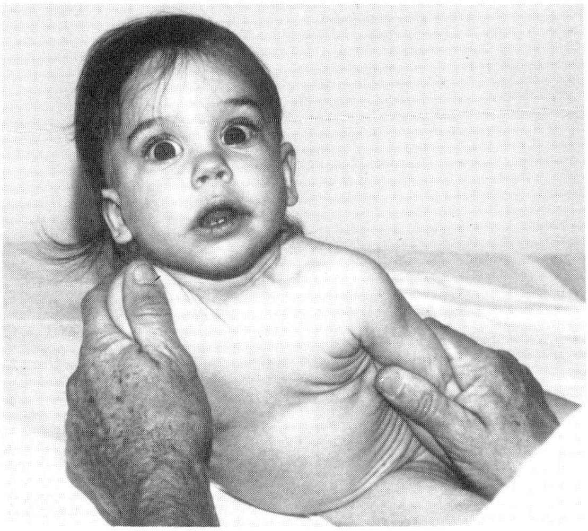

FIG. 47. Lateral abduction reaction: Lateral movements of head (control). Infant is capable of head control without additional support. Horizontal alignment of eyes is maintained when examiner inclines infant laterally.

2. If the infant cannot lift his or her head alone, the examiner must curve the trunk and support the head with one hand. While doing so, the examiner will rapidly raise and lower the neck (Figs. 48 and 49). After a series of repeated passive flexions, an active contraction of the neck will trigger the reaction.

Lateral straightening of the head is evident very soon after birth. This aspect of head control precedes and is more pronounced than is posterior straightening, (e.g., when an infant is in a sitting position), or anterior straightening, (e.g., during the pull-to-sitting maneuver). Lateral straightening is manifest only with the infant in lateral decubitus, without support to the head.

Body Support

The infant must not be allowed to relax completely or to rest in the examiner's hands. In fact, the examiner must continuously lessen support to the child. This provokes a tonicity and constant tremor in the infant, as if grasping at air during a free fall (Fig. 50). In order to produce this effect, it is suggested that the infant be placed at the edge or corner of a table with only the hip in contact with the surface. The head and trunk are suspended over the edge of the table (Fig. 51). This positioning is necessary in order to force the infant to struggle against body gravity, thereby initiating a dynamic motor response.

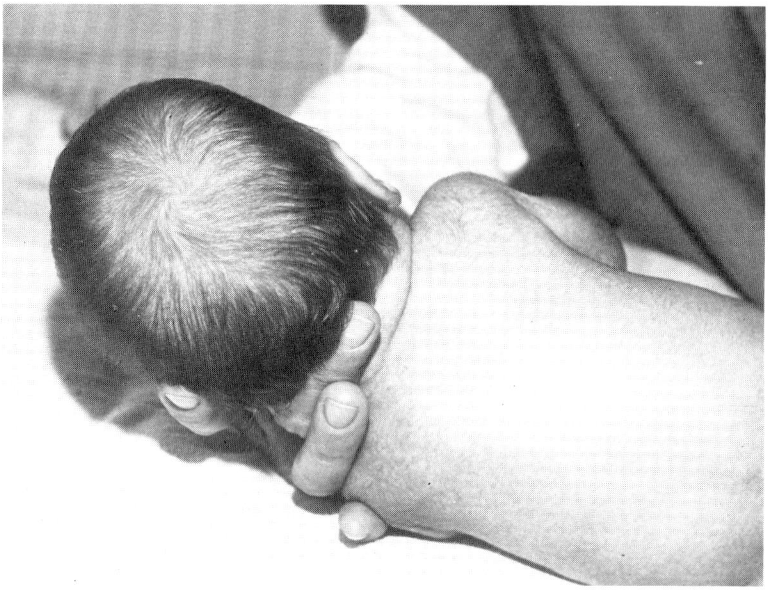

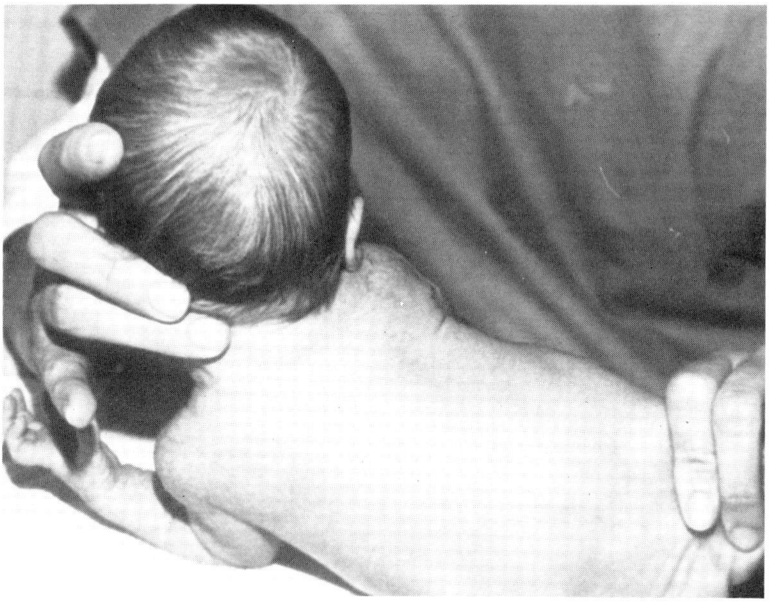

FIGS. 48 AND 49. Lateral abduction reaction: Lateral movements of head (straightening). Infant is unable to straighten head laterally. Examiner initiates series of rapid lateral straightening movements.

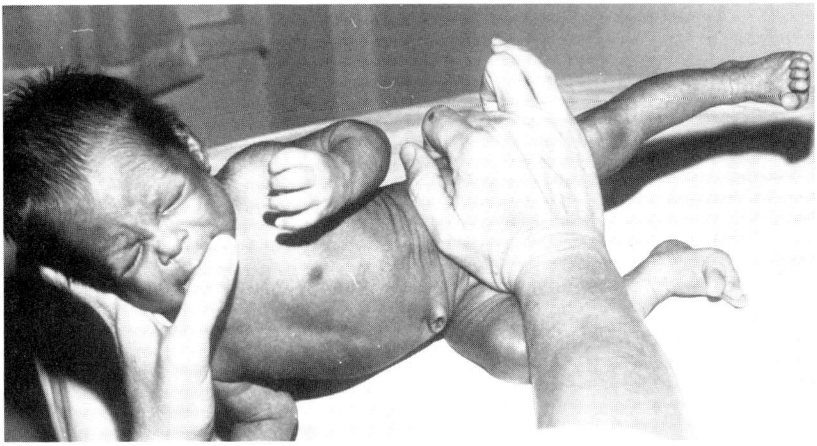

FIG. 50. Lateral abduction reaction: Support of body. Examiner suspends infant's body over examination table, thereby allowing infant to react as if falling.

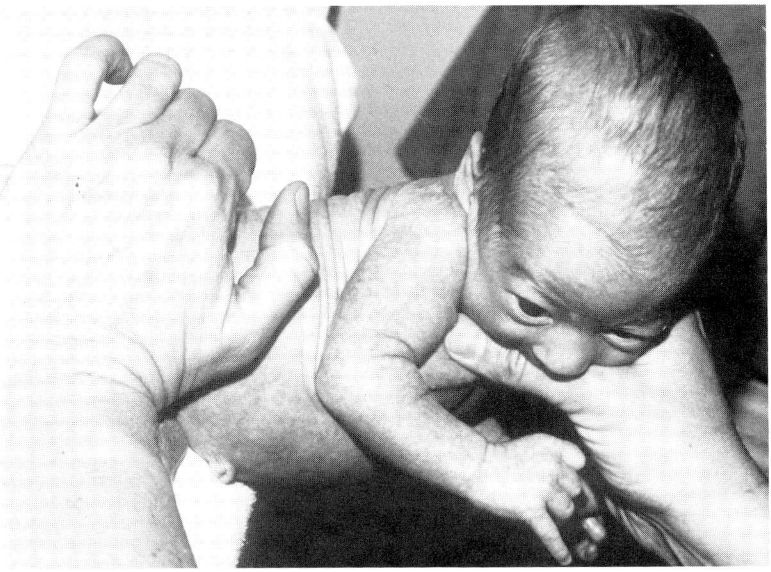

FIG. 51. Lateral abduction reaction: Support of body. Infant is positioned with body and head suspended over edge of table. Sole support point is bottom hip.

Exclusion of the Upper Extremities

The infant must not be allowed to use the hands to grasp onto the examiner or to lean on the table. Doing so would preclude all straightening efforts, thereby eliminating extension of the trunk and lower extremities.

Necessary Flexions of the Leg Resting on the Table

The limb resting on the table must be kept flexed in order to prevent its involvement in the motor response (Fig. 52). This is important for two reasons. First, this precaution distinguishes between a simple defensive extension of both limbs and the directed extension of one lower extremity, i.e., extension caused by the sudden straightening of the head. Second, maintained extension in the lower limb increases the straightening efforts to balance the body.

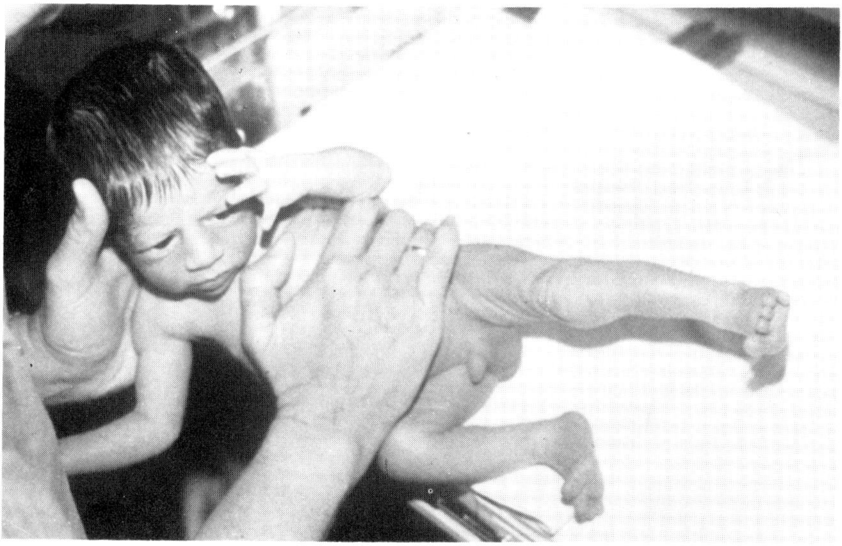

FIG. 52. Lateral abduction reaction: Flexion of "bottom" leg. This position is essential in order to avoid confusing LAR with defensive straightening of entire body.

Optimal State

As in all aspects of the neurological examination, it is essential to note certain state conditions (e.g., wakefulness, time of examination in relation to feeding, room temperature).[26,28,35] The maneuver must not be unduly distressing, although the infant may cry. Crying, in itself, is not necessarily detrimental; however, if the infant fights the procedure, the examination must be postponed until he or she is calm.

EXAMINATION TECHNIQUE (PRACTICAL APPLICATION)

We can offer some practical advice about holding the infant at the start of the maneuver and during the actual response. The suggestions depend on two factors: the infant's age and ability to manage head control.

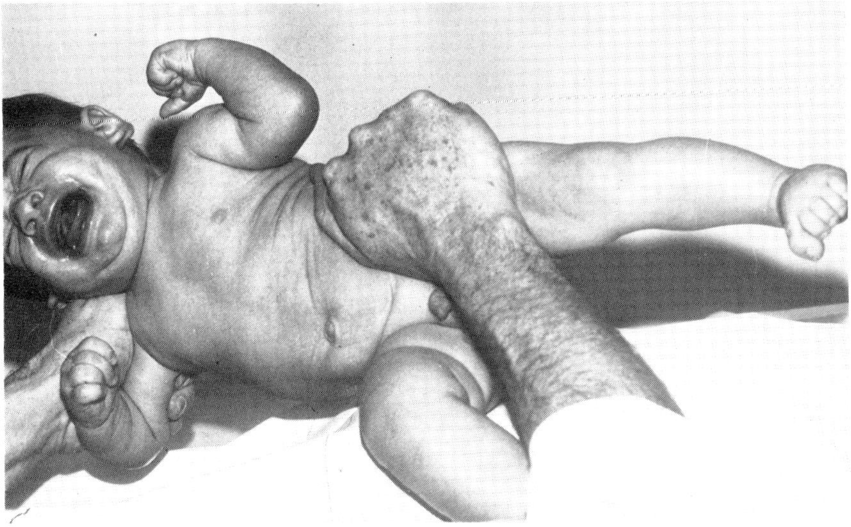

FIG. 53. Lateral abduction reaction: General conditions of examination. LAR may be present, even if infant cries.

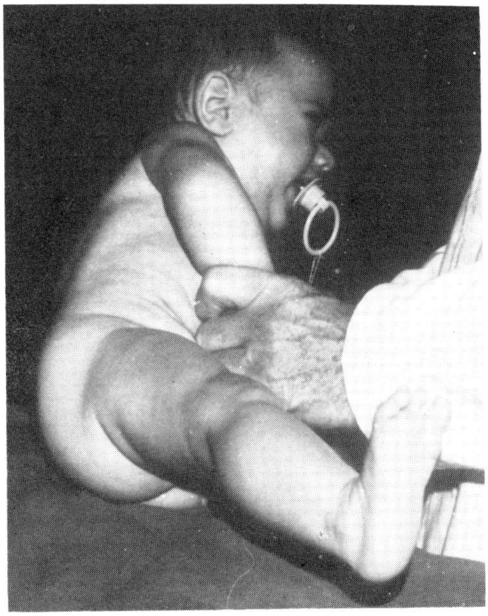

FIG. 54. Lateral abduction reaction after 6 months of age: Clinical demonstration. LAR is initiated as infant attempts to reestablish balance. Examiner grasps infant's arms and rocks body to side. Head will straighten and lower extremity will be lifted, although remaining in extension (abduction has not yet occurred).

Older Infants

If the infant is at least 6 months of age, the lateral abduction reaction can be initiated from a sitting position, with both legs hanging over the edge of the table. Because the older infant controls straightening of the head and trunk, any change in body position will provoke a balancing reaction (Fig. 54). The examiner can prevent the infant from leaning on the table by providing support under the arms. The examiner tips the infant to the side; the head straightens automatically. On the lowered side, the leg remains flexed and hooks onto the edge of the table. The opposite leg kicks forward. Only one buttock rests on the table top (Fig. 55). The infant is then pivoted toward the examiner, and the entire trunk is suspended over the edge of the table. While rotating the infant, the examiner lessens support to the infant and lets the shoulder drop somewhat. As a result of this maneuver, the extended lower extremity will abduct and protrude over the examination table. In order to assure complete abduction of the hip, the examiner may use an elbow to push the infant's knee and hip into complete extension (Figs. 56 and 57). It is important to note that the abduction is not valid unless the infant remains in a frontal orientation throughout the maneuver.

Infants Less Than 6 Months of Age

In young infants, the lateral abduction reaction is initiated from a decubitus position. The examiner must control both the head movements and the flexion in the "bottom" leg (Fig. 58). Flexion must be maintained in the leg that is not being examined. The opposite hip is held firmly in extension. At this time, the examiner must also begin the slow, lateral head movements. Because of the complexity of this maneuver, it may be advisable to work with an assistant in maintaining the body posture. Several techniques can be used to move the head laterally: 1) the examiner

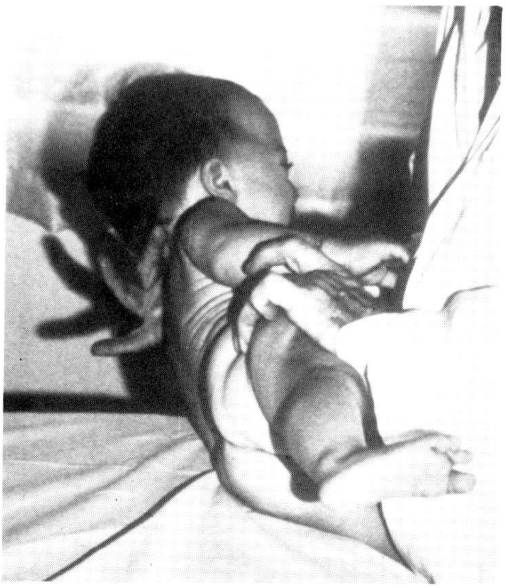

FIG. 55. Lateral abduction reaction after 6 months of age: Clinical demonstration. Abduction will occur as lower extremity is in perfect extension (ear, hip, and external malleola are aligned).

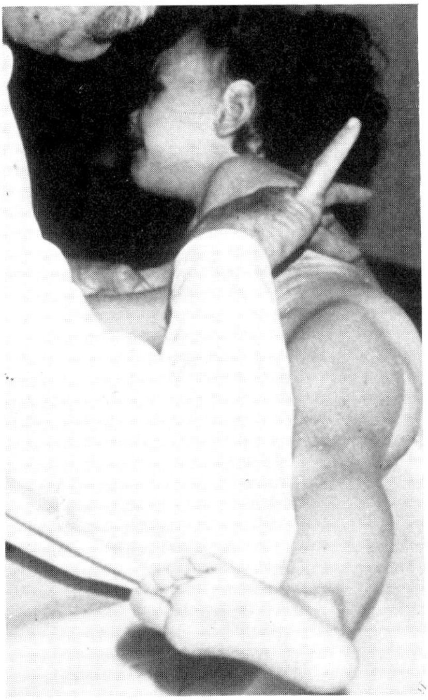

FIG. 56. Lateral abduction reaction after 6 months of age: Clinical demonstration. Trunk is suspended with lower extremity extended over table. Hip will lift and abduct as soon as examiner withdraws support. (Lower extremity is not yet aligned with trunk.)

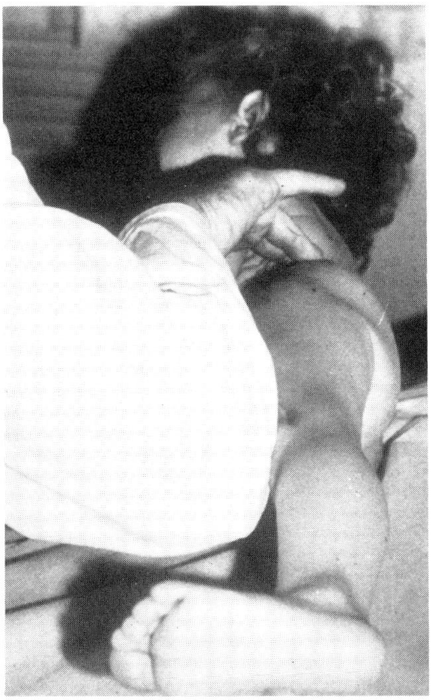

FIG. 57. Lateral abduction reaction after 6 months of age: Clinical demonstration. Alignment of lower extremity, absent in Fig. 56, is now apparent. Examiner pushes head with elbow. Both orientation of foot and abduction of hip are correct.

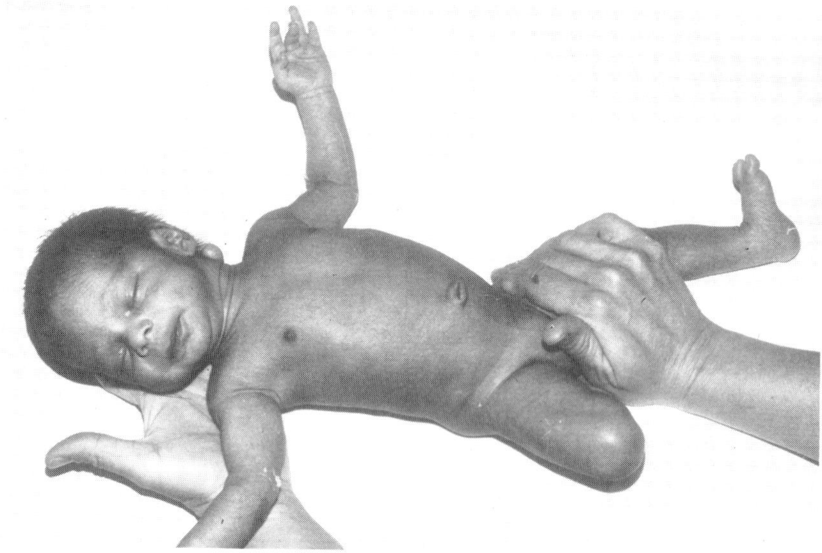

FIG. 58. Lateral abduction reaction before 6 months of age: Clinical demonstration. Examiner must control movement of head, flexion of the bottom leg, and extension of top leg.

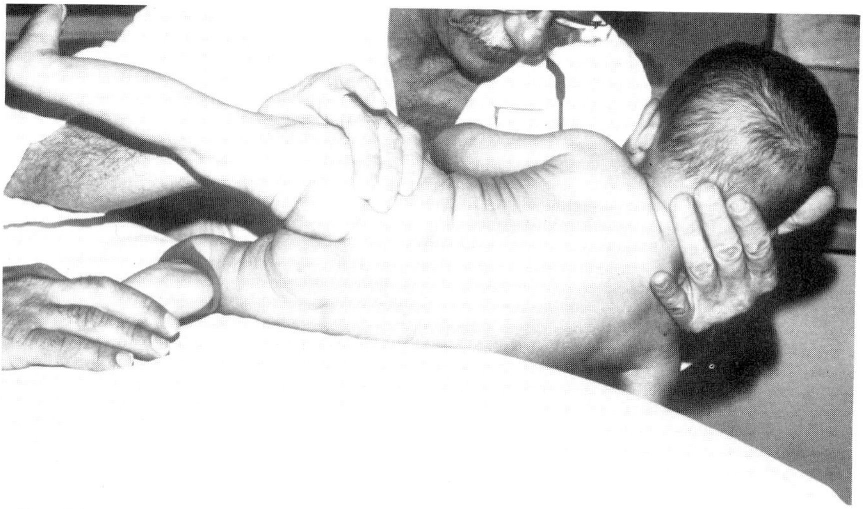

FIG. 59. Lateral abduction reaction before 6 months of age: Clinical demonstration. Examiner holds infant's cheek and ear in palm while flexing head laterally.

may move the head while supporting the infant's cheek in the palm of the hand (Fig. 59); 2) the examiner may hold the lower of the two shoulders, leaving the head suspended over the edge of the examination table while moving the head slightly up and down (Fig. 60); or 3) the examiner may

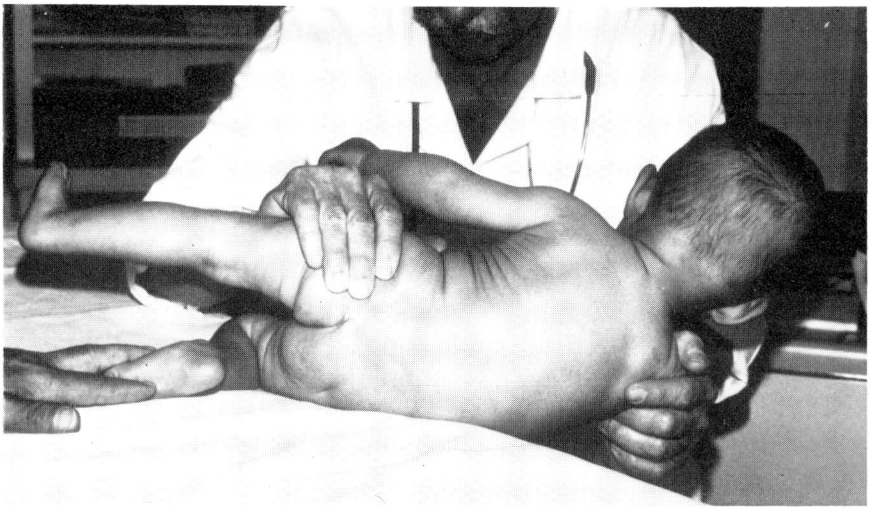

FIG. 60. Lateral abduction reaction before 6 months of age: Clinical demonstration. Examiner holds bottom shoulder, leaving head suspended over table.

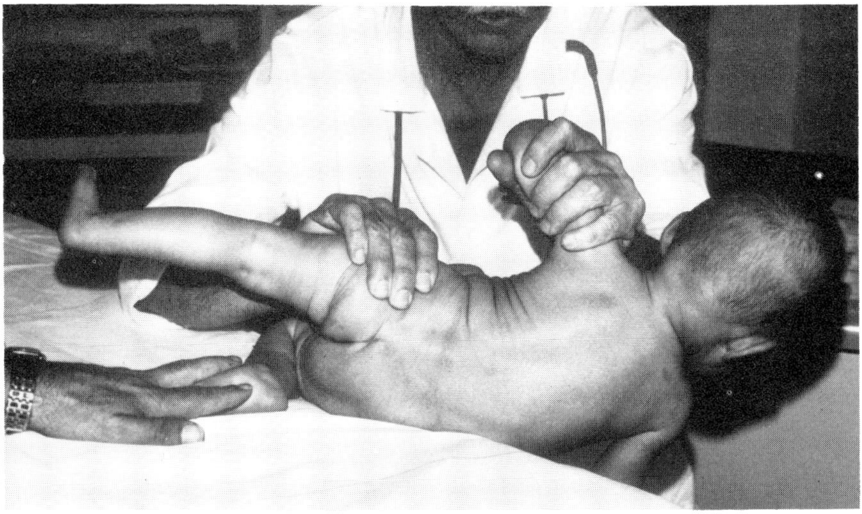

FIG. 61. Lateral abduction reaction before 6 months of age: Clinical demonstration. Examiner holds top arm, leaving head and part of trunk suspended over table.

hold onto the top arm, leaving the head, shoulder, and upper portion of the trunk suspended over the table (Fig. 61).

It can be difficult to extend the hip correctly at around the 5th or 6th month of life because of the very strong hip flexion characteristic of this age. If this is noted, an assistant might help keep the bottom leg in com-

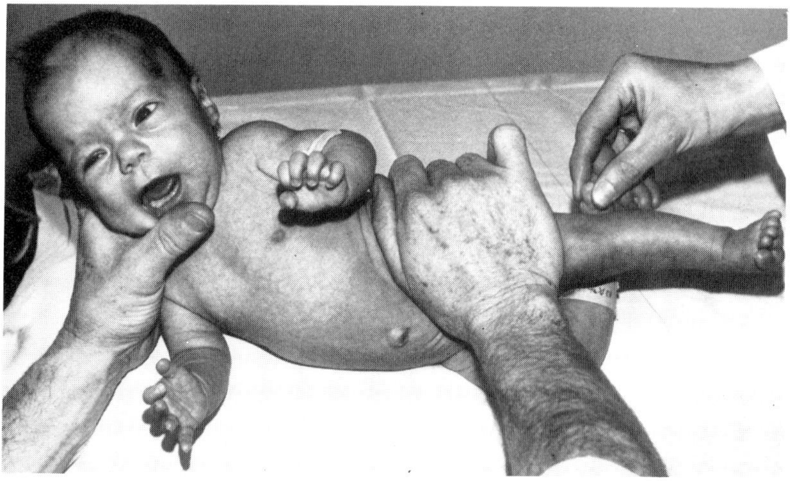

FIG. 62. Lateral abduction reaction: Clinical demonstration. Assistant may maintain flexion in bottom leg.

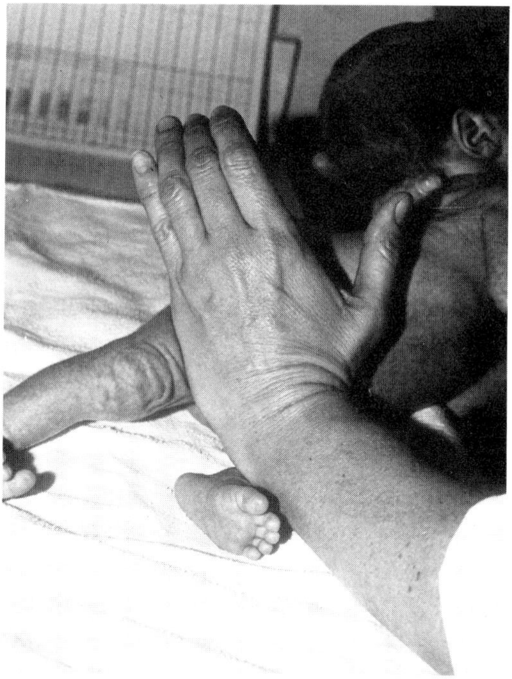

FIG. 63. Lateral abduction reaction before 6 months of age: Clinical demonstration. Examiner must push hip without force until perfect alignment is obtained.

plete flexion (Fig. 62); however, the infant must not be allowed to lean against the assistant's hand as this would invalidate the reaction. By working with an assistant, the examiner will be better able to observe the extension of the leg and hip. The examiner may push the hip to achieve a

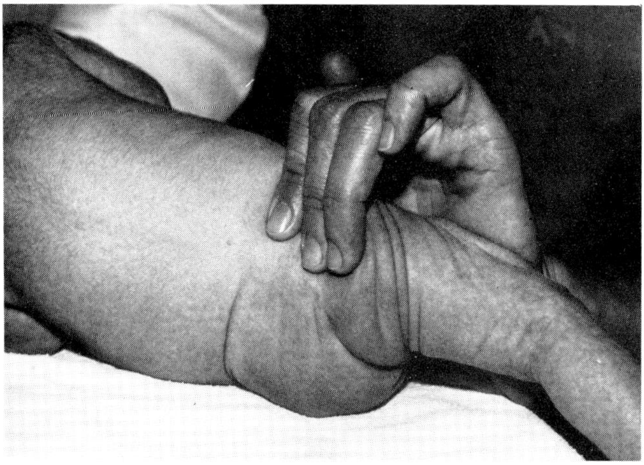

FIG. 64. Lateral abduction reaction before 6 months of age: Clinical demonstration. Examiner's hand will bridge iliac crest to create countersupport necessary to maintain hip alignment.

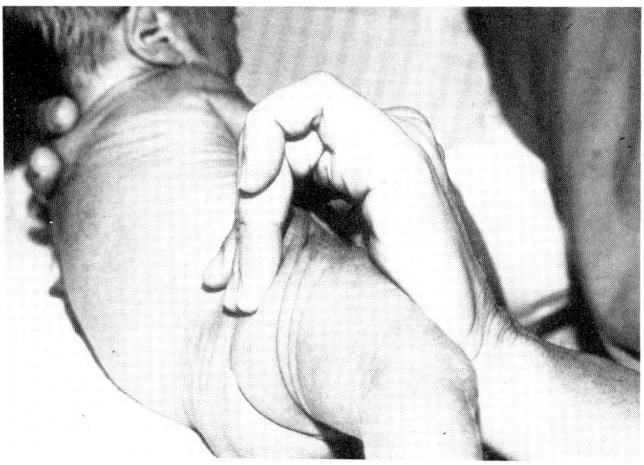

FIG. 65. Lateral abduction reaction before 6 months of age: Clinical demonstration. As examiner's fingers bridge iliac crest, they do not prevent lateral abduction of hip.

perfect alignment, but this alignment must not be forced (Fig. 63). The fingers will flex and hook behind the iliac crest as a countersupport (Figs. 64 and 65), but adequate space must be allowed for abduction of the lower extremity during the dynamic response.

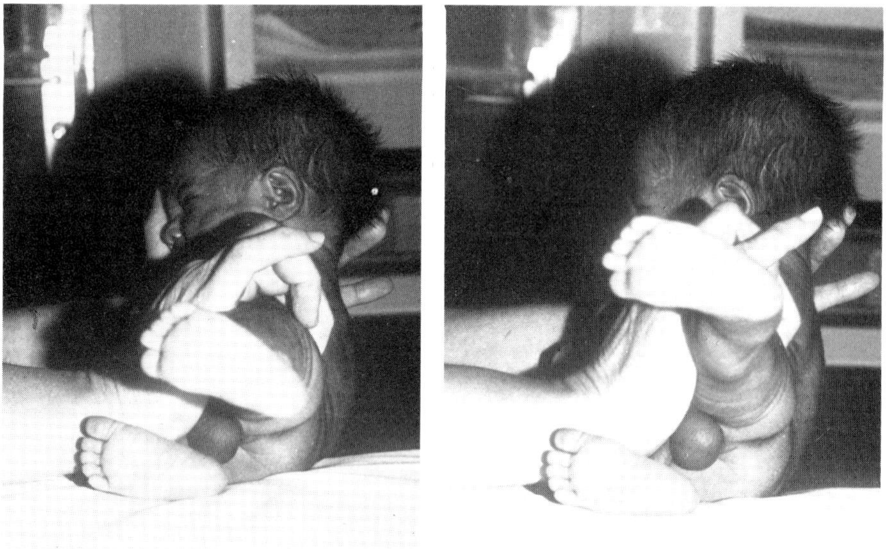

Figs. 66 and 67. Lateral abduction reaction: Dorsiflexion. Foot remains in dorsiflexion and must move up and down several times.

COMMON ERRORS IN TECHNIQUE AND INTERPRETATION

It is possible to make certain observational errors even though one might have followed all precautions and technical advice. We will not review the technical difficulties described previously, but will focus instead on problems in interpretation.

Abduction must be obvious. For example, dorsiflexion in a foot is observed as a clear and repeated flexion and extension (Figs. 66 and 67). Abduction must be verified even in those infants held by the examiner at the hip and iliac crest. Because of the significance attributed to the lateral abduction reaction, the infant's performance must not be interpreted unless the following conditions have been met: the body must not be flexed; the leg resting on the examination table must remain in flexion; the opposite extremity must be aligned perfectly, with the knee extended and the foot pointed toward the examiner. The significance of the reaction is discussed in the result section (page 82).

INDUCTION OF THE LATERAL ABDUCTION REACTION

It is actually possible to teach this reaction. Because the presence of this reaction confirms the normalcy of neuromotor function, it is appropriate to foster the reaction in the neurologically suspect newborn or young infant. It is preferable that this investigation be carried out by an occupational therapist with specialized training in the exercise of this reaction. Importantly, however, the goal is not to construct the reaction artificially by imposing acrobatic positions. As the chain reaction that produces contractions along the side of the body is present from birth, it is sufficient to bring together the motor conditions necessary for clinical expression of the response.

The process initially stimulates and strengthens the infant's efforts to straighten the head. This effort is followed by a straightening of that portion of the trunk resting on the upper extremity. The examiner rolls the infant from the back to the side by pushing against the hip (Fig. 68). The infant's movements are counterbalanced by the examiner in order to maintain the position as long as possible (Fig. 69). Gradually, the infant will learn to straighten the upper portion of the trunk and to support the trunk with the elbow. The examiner should not pull on the top arm during this maneuver.

Only after the infant's head has lifted from the table should the examiner pull on the arms to reinforce the lower trunk and to align the head and trunk (Fig. 70). Mild traction is applied to the shoulders after the head has been lifted and straightened laterally (Fig. 71). At this point, the infant will more spontaneously use the elbow, forearm, or even a hand for support. Because perfect alignment between the head and trunk is essential during these maneuvers, the infant must not be allowed to turn toward the examiner (Fig. 72).

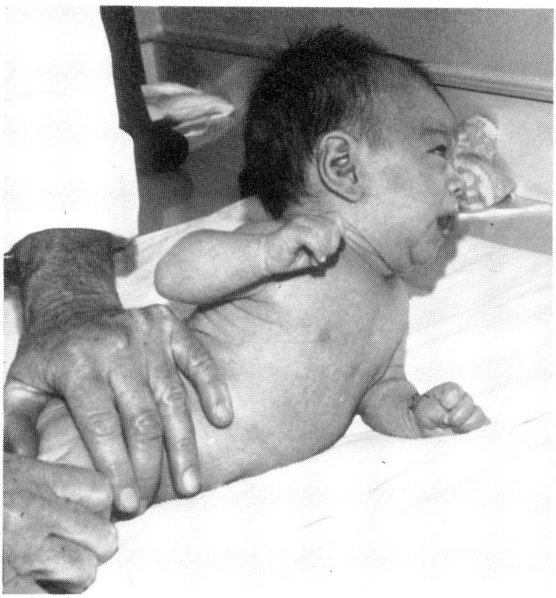

FIG. 68. Induction of lateral abduction reaction (J10). Straightening is apparent in head and upper portion of trunk. Infant is supported by bottom arm. Examiner then rolls infant onto his hip, maintaining infant balanced on one flank.

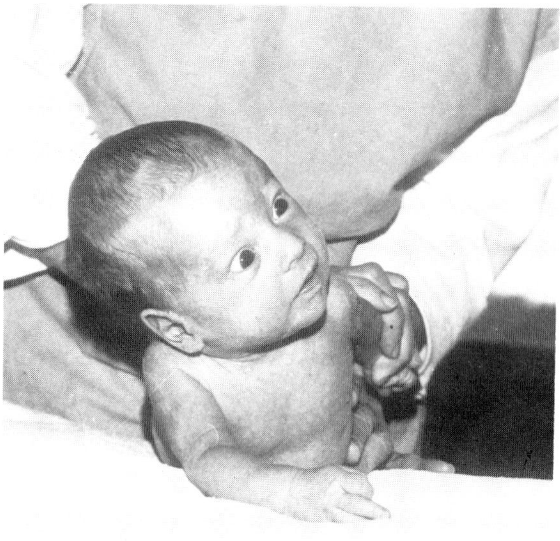

FIG. 69. Induction of lateral abduction reaction (J10). Note straightening of head and of upper portion of trunk. Examiner counterbalances rocking of head and trunk.

The frequency of these "training sessions" should be dictated by the infant's needs. More frequent exercise sessions would be indicated in infants manifesting neurological abnormalities. If a pathological situation should develop, accelerated postural regulation and more intensive physical rehabilitation should be attempted. Postural regulation can be improved. Lateral abduction reaction therapy has been effective in correcting both abnormalities in posture and motor activities. It should be recognized, however, that these inductive maneuvers are more dependent on optimal environmental factors than the routine neurological examination. The infant must be cooperative and undistracted.

It is important that the infant not be unduly upset by these manipulations. Afferent stimuli soon cause the infant to stiffen and struggle; however, the effects of these stimuli can be reduced by careful monitoring of the speed, force, and amplitude of the muscle manipulations. If this is not respected, contractions will be exaggerated and motor reactions may be either misdirected or absent. One must avoid brusque stimuli that might startle the infant or cause crying, thereby interrupting the motor sequence. Before initiating the directed movements, it is advisable to grasp the muscles firmly and to begin with small movements that would achieve relaxation.

Swinging of the head represents yet another source of afferent stimuli, especially during the first 3 months of life. At this age, head control is quite unstable and these involuntary movements may be large and rapid. This instability may cause the infant to stiffen and become uncooperative. Examination would be impossible. Although the head is not supported

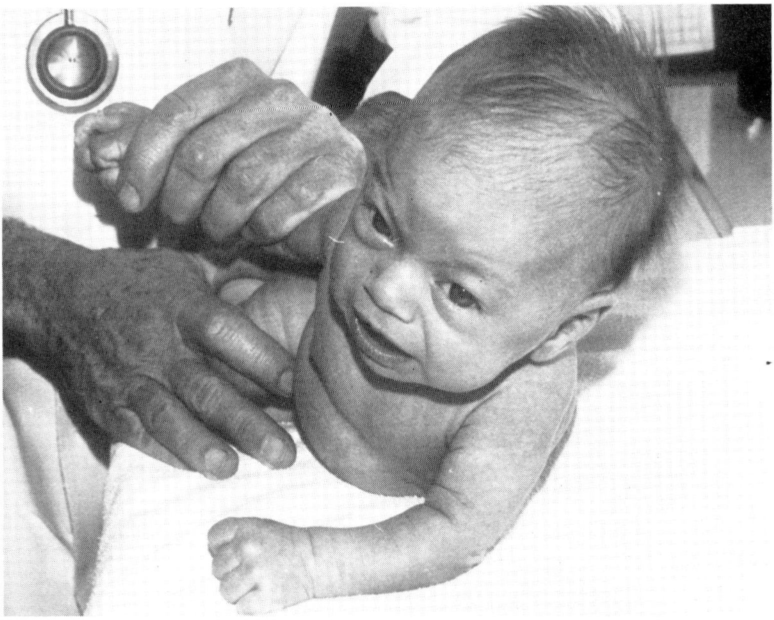

FIG. 70. Induction of the lateral abduction reaction (J20). Examiner reinforces alignment of head and trunk. Maneuver is initiated by exerting traction on arm.

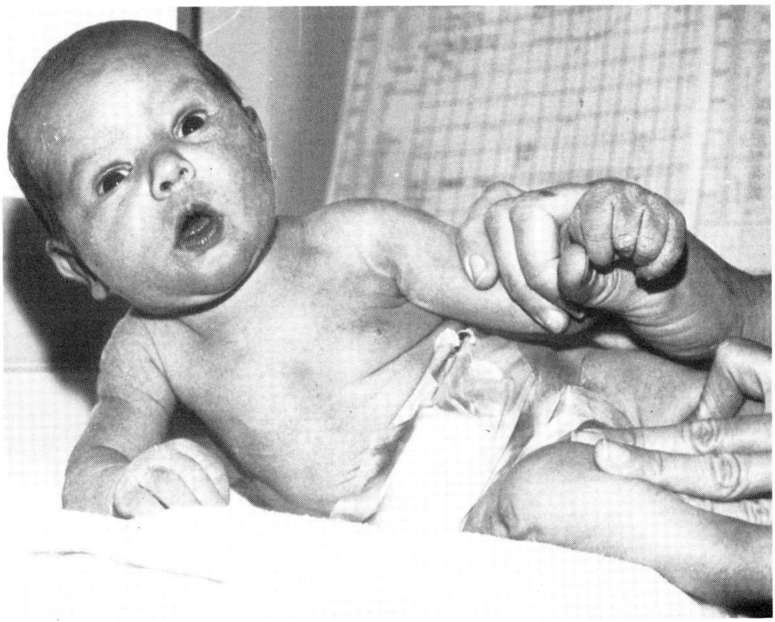

FIG. 71. Lateral abduction reaction (J5). Head has already lifted. Examiner encourages reaction by exerting mild traction on shoulder.

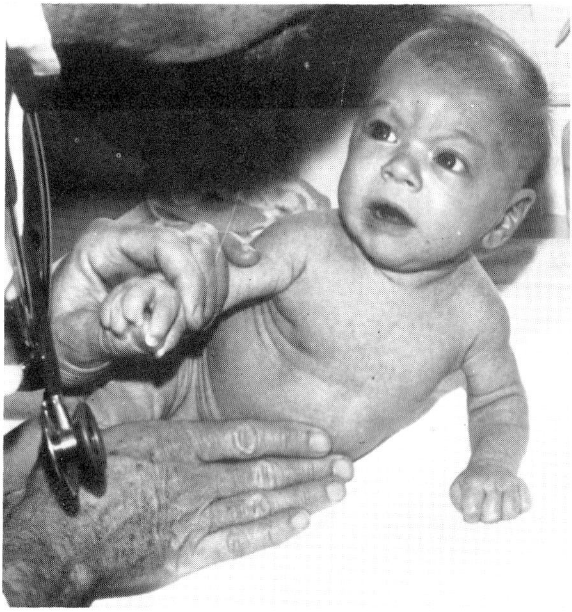

FIG. 72. Induction of the lateral abduction reaction. In order to reinforce lateral straightening of trunk, infant must be prevented from turning head to look at examiner.

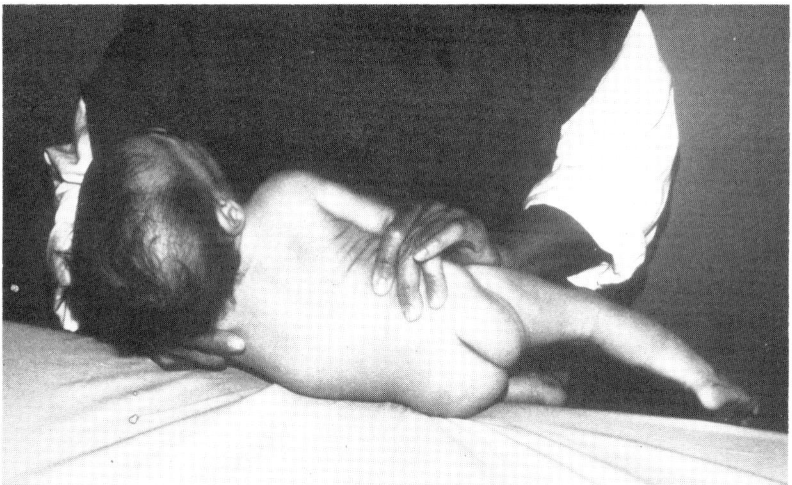

FIG. 73. Lateral abduction reaction indications: Infant with cerebral palsy. Motor chain reaction is disturbed. LAR is absent.

during the exercise for induction of the lateral abduction reaction, one can guard against any unexpected movements between maneuvers by supporting the head and moving the infant smoothly from the sitting to decubitus position.

TABLE 4
Principal Risk Conditions in 419 Neonatal Observations

Risk Categories	*Number of Cases*
Prematurity	96
Icterus and exchange transfusion	39
Neurological distress	61
Respiratory distress	55
Small for gestational age	51
Severe acute dehydration	42
Severe infection	18
Unclassified	57
Total	419

TABLE 5
Principal Neurological Anomalies in 419 Neonatal Observations

Risk Categories	*Number of Cases*
Hypotonia	87
Hypertonia	66
Modified primary reflexes	20
Hyperexcitability	14
Decreased postural regulation	38
Asymmetry	17
Poor psychobehavorial alertness	25
Unclassified	152
Total	419

TABLE 6
Results of the Study of the Lateral Abduction Reaction in 419 Cases–Neurological Status at Age 1 Year and Older in Relationship to the Absence or Presence of the Reaction[a]

LAR	*Number of Cases*	*Neurological Status at 1 yr Age or Older*
Absent	35	18 CP 17 Non-CP
Present	384	384 Non-CP
Total	419	

[a]LAR, lateral with abduction reaction; CP, cerebral palsy.

INDICATIONS AND RATIONALE FOR CONTINUED STUDY OF THE LATERAL ABDUCTION REACTION

As reported by Vojta,[37] the directed motor sequence is always abnormal in infants with cerebral palsy (Fig. 73). We also know that abnormal hip abduction in these infants is common very early in life. The lateral abduction reaction is a dynamic motor maneuver capable of assessing both anomalies.

Indications for the maneuver were changed by evidence of absent lateral abduction reaction in pathological situations other than cerebral palsy. Our research indicates that the presence of a normal lateral abduction reaction is a sign of neuromotor integrity. Absence of the lateral abduction reaction is not necessarily an early indication of cerebral palsy; however, presence of the reaction allows us to eliminate that diagnosis.

Of course, this finding has broadened the indications for carrying out the maneuver. The lateral abduction reaction has an important prognostic value in relationship to cerebral palsy well before suspect infants are able to stand or walk. The maneuver also represents an important component of the neuromotor examination during the first 3 months of life. Indeed, during this period, a normal bilateral reaction confirms normal neuromotor function and predicts subsequent neuromotor integrity.

We are now performing this maneuver routinely during the neurological examination and are currently comparing performance in normal and at-risk infant populations in our perinatal center.

STUDY FINDINGS

Two questions are prompted by the following findings from a study including at-risk newborns: Is it possible to confirm developmental prognosis and to rule out a diagnosis of cerebral palsy during the 1st year of life? Will the lateral abduction reaction provide motor prognosis before 3 months of age?

Study Population

At-risk newborns were examined at birth and through the 1st year of life, or until each infant began to walk. The study was carried out by one medical team. Of the 546 infants enrolled in the study, 127 were eliminated, 88 were lost to follow-up, and 39 were not followed throughout the entire study period. The 419 remaining infants are included in the present study findings.

Primary risk factors are described in Table 4 and were recorded for each examination. If no risk factor was found to predominate, the observation was recorded under Other. All infants had one or more transient neurological abnormalities (Table 5). However, if no single anomaly predominated, this also was recorded under Other. The findings report the most significant anomaly for each infant during the first 2 months of life.

Absence of the Lateral Abduction Reaction

In 35 infants, the lateral abduction reaction was absent throughout all developmental stages (Table 6). Of these infants, cerebral palsy developed in 18 and did not develop in 17. The lateral abduction reaction was observed in 384 infants, none of whom developed cerebral palsy. Although the reaction appeared at various developmental stages, once confirmed, the reaction remained present.

Table 7 provides outcome summaries for those 35 infants in whom a lateral abduction reaction failed to develop. In 18 infants, i.e., 4.6% of the study population, cerebral palsy developed. Although early physical therapy was initiated in 13 infants, 8 of whom were enrolled in the treatment program during the 1st month of life, no improvement in cerebral palsy was noted in any of these infants. The most frequently observed clinical syndrome was dyskinetic–dystonia (13 cases).

Cerebral palsy did not develop in 17 of the infants who were free of CNS anomalies on follow-up (Table 7). The following factors were attributed to the absent lateral abduction reaction among these 17 infants: hip dysplasia (6 cases); subdural hematoma with complete recovery and without motor sequellae after drainage (4 cases); and unknown cause (7 cases).

Presence of the Lateral Abduction Reaction

No signs of cerebral palsy were found in 384 infants. All have had normal neuromotor development. Because these infants have not been re-

TABLE 7
Details of 35 Cases with Absent Lateral Abduction Reaction[a]

LAR Absent	*Number of Cases*	*Development*	
		Cause	*N*
CP	18	Spastic diplegia	3
		Dyskinetic dystonia	13
		Hemiplegia	2
Non-CP	17	Dysplasia	6
		Subdural hematoma	4
		Unknown cause	7
Total	35		

[a]CP, cerebral palsy.

TABLE 8
Distribution of 384 Cases According to Age at Demonstration of the Lateral Abduction Reaction

	Cases		Early Prognosis	
LAR	*N*	*%*	*N*	*%*
1st month	132	34.3	–	–
1–3 months	128	33.4	260	68
After 3 months	124	32.3	–	–
Total	384	100	–	–

examined on follow-up by either a medical or psychological team, a complete intellectual and sensory evaluation is not included in this report.

The lateral abduction reaction is not always evidenced during the first several months of life. If we eliminate those cases in which the reaction appeared late, it is possible to predict normal neuromotor development in 260, i.e., 68% of the study cases by the end of the third month (Table 8).

Although early neuromotor prognosis has been correlated with transient neurological anomalies during the 1st trimester, we have not found a significant correlation between any specific neuromotor sign and difficult or delayed demonstration of the lateral abduction reaction.

Clinical Significance of the Lateral Abduction Reaction

Several conclusions can be drawn from the study findings. Presence of the lateral abduction reaction on both sides of the body precludes the risk for cerebral palsy. The lateral abduction reaction may be present as early as the first few days of life. If present, it is possible to make a motor prognosis by the end of the 3rd month of life.

Once the lateral abduction reaction has been confirmed, it is considered to be present even if difficult to demonstrate on subsequent examinations. A study of normal population has shown that if the lateral abduction reaction is to appear, it will be present by the end of the 8th month of life. After this age, absence of the reaction is prognostically significant.

Absence of the lateral abduction reaction in itself does not confirm the diagnosis of cerebral palsy. It is not unusual to encounter great difficulty in demonstrating the lateral abduction reaction. Our experience has suggested several explanations for this difficulty. Lack of examiner confidence is a common factor. If an otherwise neurologically normal infant refuses to participate in the examination, the response is considered absent. No practical conclusions can be drawn in this instance.

Decreased extensibility of the hip flexor muscles may also complicate the examination, especially in an infant between ages 3–6 months. Hypertonicity resulting from decreased extensibility is exaggerated by any attempt to stretch the muscles. A similar situation is created in the first 4 months of life if the infant is diapered in a position of abduction. If the hips are rotated externally and maintained in flexion, it is difficult to modify the position by passive mobilization. The muscles behave as if they were shortened and will resist any stretching maneuver.

Such difficulties are also encountered in infants who are usually kept lying on their abdomen. Lifting the head flexes the trunk and maintains the lower extremities in external rotation. Alignment of the neck, head, and trunk becomes difficult. Even if the lower extremities can be extended correctly, those infants frequently remain in their preferred position of external rotation. Correct response is not possible if the foot is directed upward with the lower extremity elevated, i.e., elevation of the lower extremity is produced by the flexor and not the abductor muscles.

Absence of a lateral abduction reaction may be attributable to skeletal, joint, or muscle abnormalities unrelated to CNS anomalies. This possibility must be considered in infants at risk for neurological anomalies, as well as in those infants having an otherwise normal examination. In several cases, the absence of the lateral abduction reaction was attributable to hip dysplasia. This finding is especially relevant during the first 4 months of life, during which time it is difficult to evaluate the orthopedic function of the hip by either clinical or radiological techniques. In six observations (reported earlier), dormant articular abnormalities were suspected because of an abnormal lateral abduction reaction. In these cases, no other signs were present. Hip dysplasia was later confirmed radiologically. Moreover, we have learned that 1) any pathology of the hip can interfere with the lateral abduction reaction; and 2) the reaction is never expressed when subluxation or luxation of the hip is diagnosed clinically or radiologically. An absent lateral abduction reaction is consistent with osteoarthritis and has contributed frequently to the diagnosis of other disease in the hip.

It is more difficult to understand the correlation between the absence of a lateral abduction reaction and a subdural hematoma. In four infants with subdural hematomas treated by repeated aspiration, the lateral abduction reaction did not appear until after complete resolution of the condition. The reaction appeared concurrent with normal transillumination. Interestingly, the hematoma was always localized on the side of the body without lateral abduction, i.e., the relationship between the abnormal reaction and hematoma was ipsilateral rather than contralateral, as expected in an injury to the CNS.

Chapter 5

Expression of Liberated Motor Activity (LMA) Following Manual Immobilization of the Head

Certain aspects of the newborn's complex motor potentials are not exhibited spontaneously, i.e., the lateral abduction reaction. We have learned that the motor activity of the newborn is dominated entirely by lack of control of the neck muscles. If the examiner artificially corrects this weakness for several minutes, motor potentials seen in older infants become evident. These motor potentialities, which we refer to as liberated motor activity, are of great theoretical interest. However, three fundamental questions must be addressed before these maneuvers can be included as an integral part of the complementary neuromotor examination of the newborn:

1. Is the absence of liberated motor activity of any prognostic value?
2. Can the presence of liberated motor activity be used to confirm normalcy at a very early age?
3. Will the repetition of these maneuvers modify the classic motor examination of the newborn?

METHODS

The liberated motor activity can be seen only during the first 2 months of life. Indeed, it is only at this age that uncontrolled head movements result in the afferent stimuli provoking obligatory responses (Fig. 74). By immobilizing the neck of an infant placed in a sitting position, uncontrolled head movements and the obligatory reactions to those movements

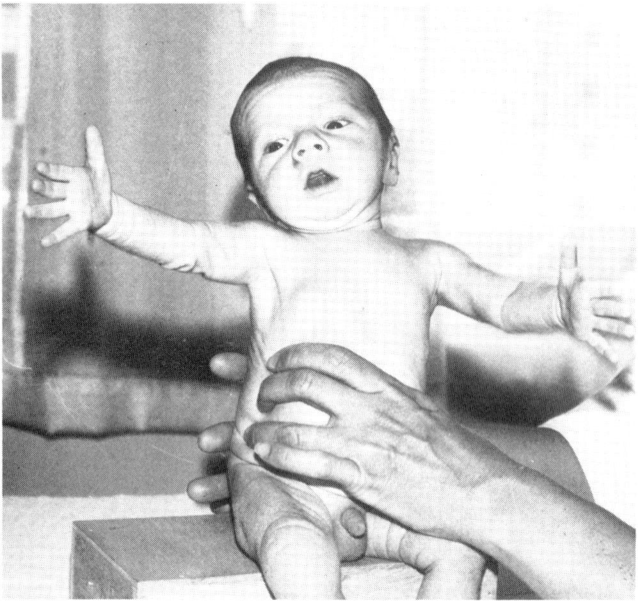

FIG. 74. Liberated motor activity: Uncontrolled movements of head initiate obligatory responses.

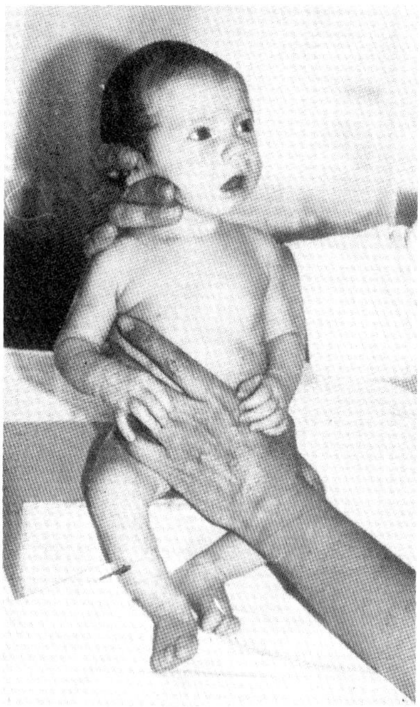

FIG. 75. Liberated motor activity: Manual immobilization of neck results in motor relaxation.

will be suppressed. The resulting calm in motor activity is prerequisite to carrying out the maneuvers described in this study (Fig. 75). Once free of any obligatory responses, the infant is able to express those motor behaviors termed liberated motor activity.

Demonstration of Liberated Motor Activity

The liberated motor activity (LMA) is set in motion after a period usually not longer than 5–6 min. During this time, the newborn will maintain a level of activity similar to that seen when the head is unsupported. The calming effect is progressive. Total relaxation must be obtained before interpreting the effects on wakefulness, resting tone of the extremities and the trunk, movements of the upper extremities, and postural tone of

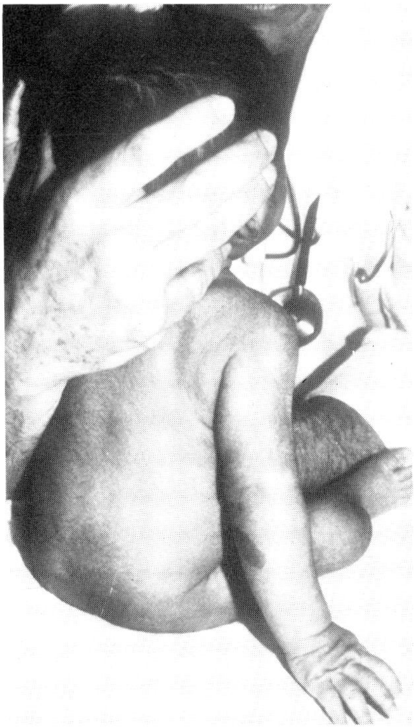

FIG. 76. Liberated motor activity: Starting position (J10). Examiner holds infant's neck and head firmly with one hand. Examiner's elbow is placed on table.

the trunk. Some of these effects can be observed in a newborn infant without specific immobilization of the head and neck, e.g., most frequently with regard to wakefulness.[1,28] These spontaneously observed responses are recorded as isolated findings noted by chance during the neurological examination. Our methodology is unique in that the effects of the LMA can be fostered and studied at will.

The examiner must both obtain and sustain motor calm throughout the entire maneuver while concurrently creating the optimal conditions

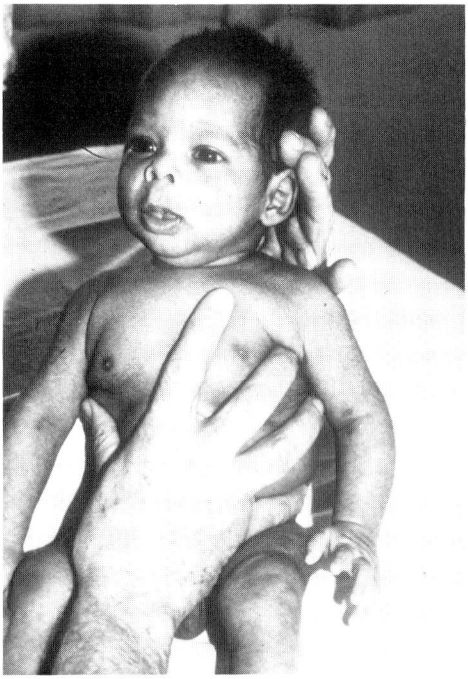

FIG. 77. Liberated motor activity: Starting position (J18). Examiner provides countersupport by placing one hand on infant's abdomen.

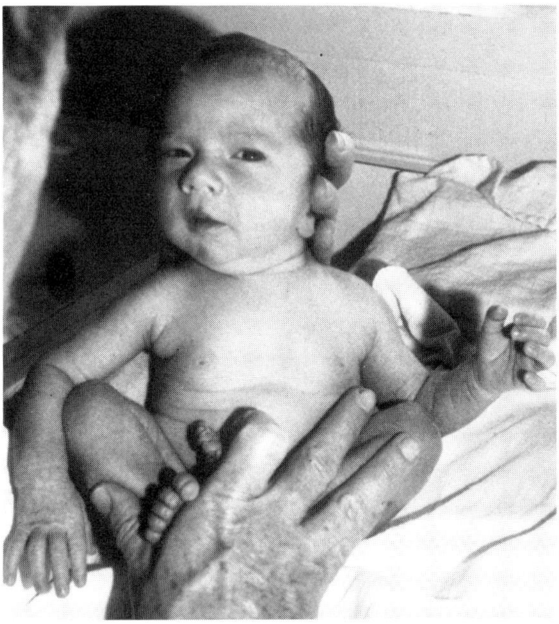

FIG. 78. Liberated motor activity: Starting position (J8). Examiner brings both legs together in flexed position. Short flexion movements are repeated.

for expression of the new motor potential. The detailed description of this technique that follows includes the development of the LMA, special precautions, and practical demonstration of the LMA. The newborn's position must be changed three times during the maneuver: 1) the infant is seated on the examination table; 2) on a bench; and 3) behind a small desk.

Starting Position

The infant is placed in a semisitting position directly in front of the examiner (Fig. 76). The examiner must control the infant's head by placing one hand behind the neck. It is essential to wait until the infant is calm

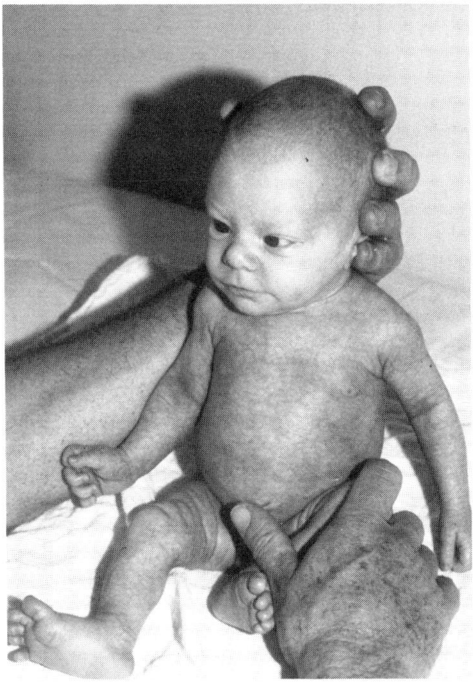

FIG. 79. Liberated motor activity: Starting position (J12). Interaction and communication with infant can be produced at will.

and attentive before bringing the infant to a full sitting position. This must be done slowly and without any abrupt change in posture. The examiner's hand is moved slowly behind the head to hold the temporal prominences on either side. The examiner's elbow rests firmly on the table with the forearm behind the infant's shoulder. The infant's back remains unsupported.

If a newborn has a tendency to fall forward, the examiner must place one hand on the infant's abdomen in order to provide additional support (Fig. 77). The examiner's thumb may be placed under the chin in order to redirect the head and prevent it from dropping forward. If the infant is moving the lower extremities, the examiner brings both legs together in a flexed position. Short flexion movements are repeated to relax the lower extremities (Fig. 78); however, this simultaneous support of the head and trunk must not immobilize the infant completely. Support should not be resisted by the infant. It is provided only to the neck muscles to promote harmonious low-amplitude movements of constant velocity. In order to achieve the appropriate motor behaviors, the examiner's hand must maintain a tremorlike movement. We also recommend moving the head up and down in a pistonlike motion; however, this movement must not be so significant as to stimulate obligatory responses.

The onset of the LMA can be observed at this point. These initial effects must be noted before proceeding with the examination. The initial effects become apparent after 3–5 min, during which time the examiner must gain and maintain the infant's visual attention. Moreover, the examiner should talk constantly to the infant, using words and sounds that will not interfere with the examination.

Initially, the infant will fight the support given by the examiner and may exhibit some jerking movements, e.g., pushing the head backward and thrusting the trunk forward. The level of alertness will change suddenly from state 2 to state 5 without apparent reason; however, this situation does not last very long, and the infant will become more and more interested in the examiner. The infant's state does not resemble any of those described by Prechtl. We refer to this level of alertness as the communication state because the infant does, indeed, communicate with the examiner (Fig. 79). Typically, the infant will look at the examiner, as if

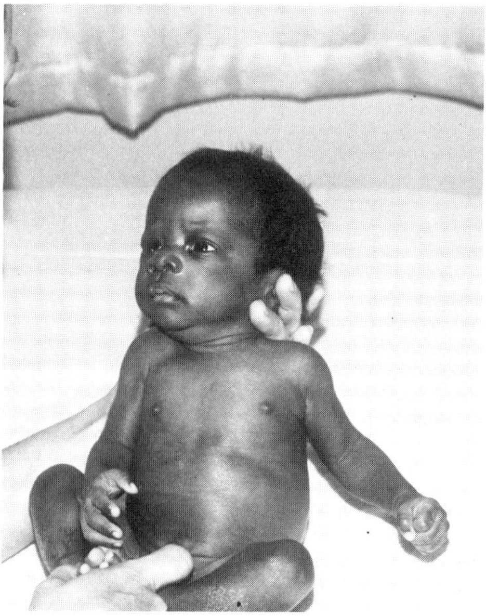

FIG. 80. Liberated motor activity: Starting position (J18). Communication state.

charmed. The infant listens attentively, makes efforts to respond, and seems to smile, as evidenced by changes in the facial expression (Figs. 80 and 81).[28]

The constant obligatory movements in the upper extremities will stop as the infant's behavior changes. Initially, the arms are raised shoulder

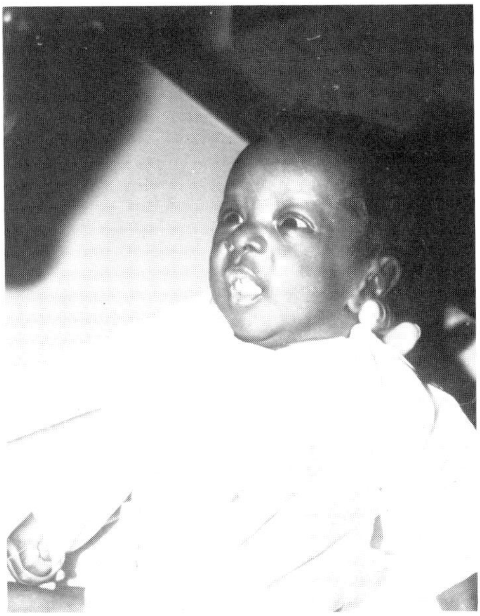

FIG. 81. Liberated motor activity: Starting position (J20). Communication state.

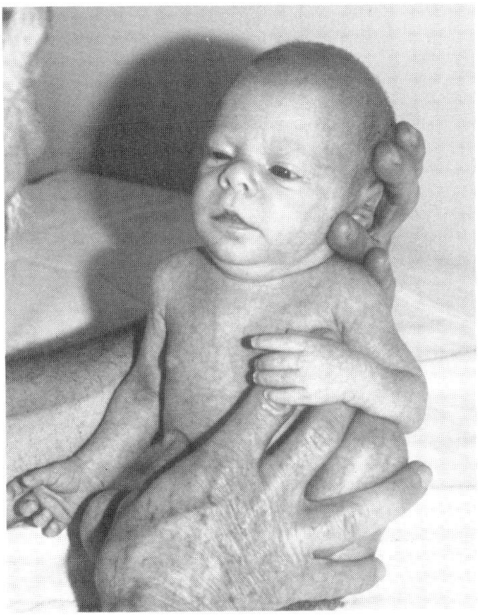

FIG. 82. Liberated motor activity: Starting position (J12). Infant's upper extremities are relaxed; hands are open.

high in response to the slightest stimulation. Gradually, these movements will weaken and become less frequent. Soon after, the infant's arms will relax and rest beside the trunk (Fig. 82). The resting tone, which decreases dramatically, resembles that of an older infant.

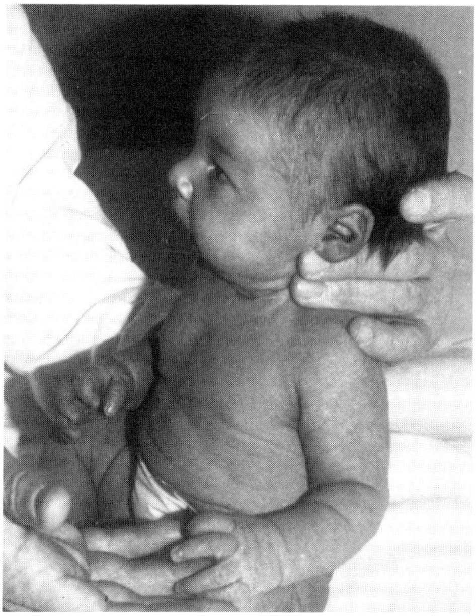

FIG. 83. Liberated motor activity: Starting position (J7). Infant's hands are open. Examiner can move last four fingers easily without resistance from infant.

During this initial period, which signals the onset of the liberated motor activity, the hands will remain partially open. The fingers are spread with only the thumb flexed across the palm (Fig. 83). Finally, without specific stimuli, some spontaneous movements will become apparent (Figs. 84 and 85). These are small, low-amplitude gestures, but appear very harmonious and coordinated, resembling natural movements of older infants.

The LMA continues to unfold and will be manifest more clearly once set in motion. It is therefore important to support the head continuously in order to avoid obligatory responses that would interrupt the necessary motor calm. We can proceed to the next step only after this state is well established. This step liberates the motor activity and promotes better observational conditions.

Observational Situation Using the Small Bench

The infant is seated on an appropriate-sized bench. The infant's thighs should be parallel to the table with the feet resting on the examination table (Fig. 86). The examiner, seated slightly to the side of the infant, continues to hold the infant's head and will look away from time to time,

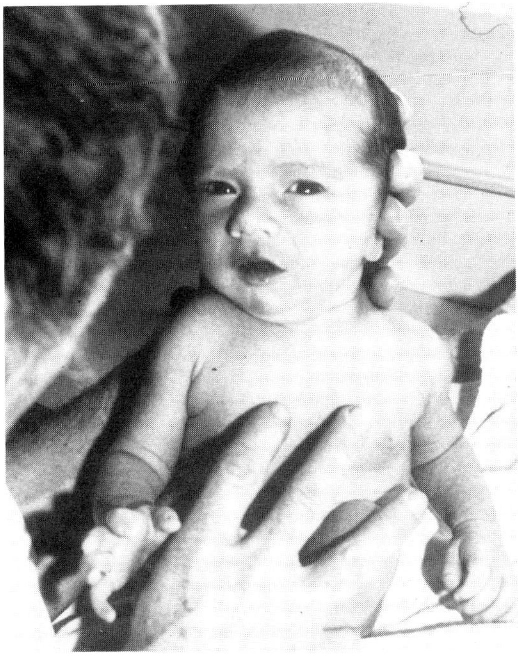

FIG. 84. Liberated motor activity: Starting position (J8). Some spontaneous movements are observed.

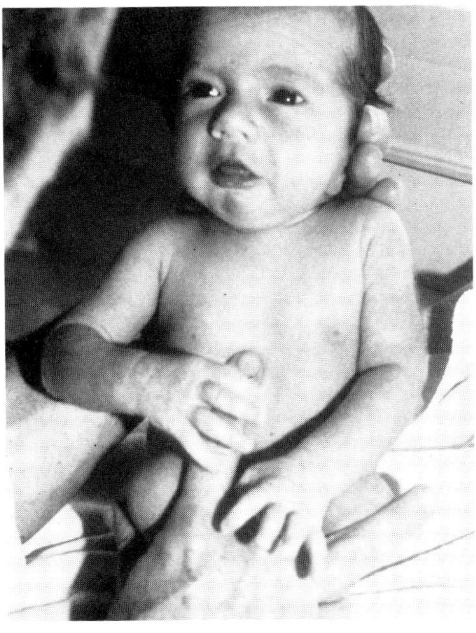

FIG. 85. Liberated motor activity: Starting position (J8). Infant manipulates examiner's fingers. Movements are similar to those seen in older infants.

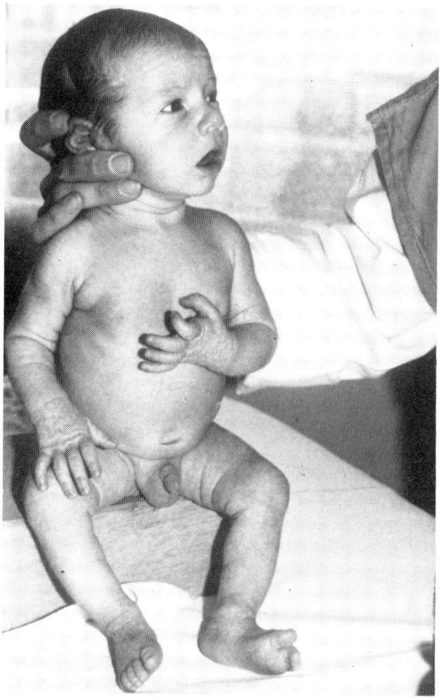

FIG. 86. Liberated motor activity: Second observational situation (J16). Infant is seated on appropriate-size bench.

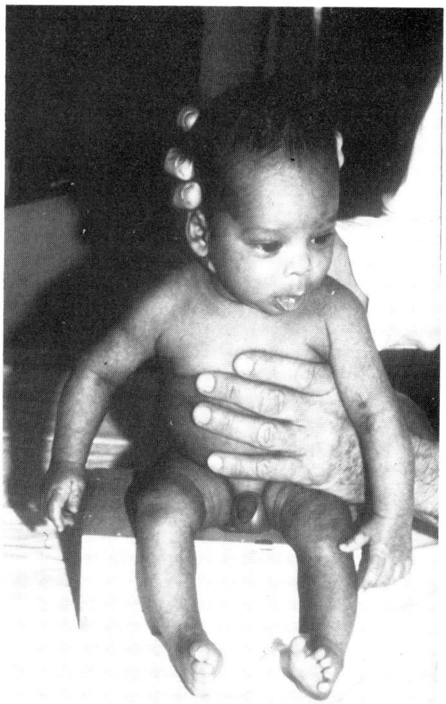

FIG. 87. Liberated motor activity: Second observational situation (J30). Examiner is seated toward side of infant. Infant does not look directly at examiner.

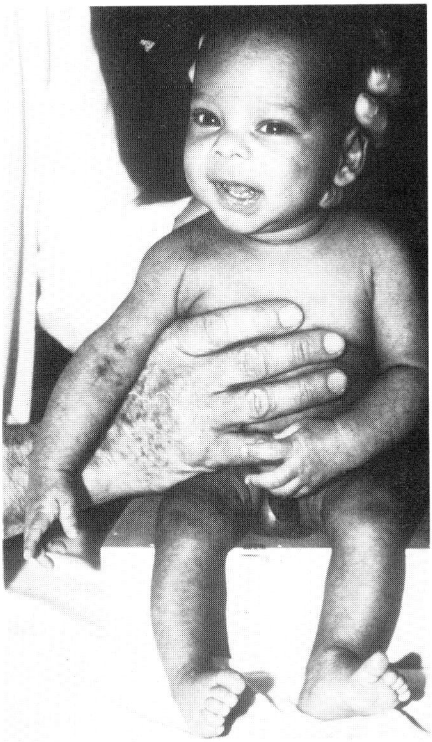

FIG. 88. Liberated motor activity: Second observational situation (J30). Hands are wide open and can move freely.

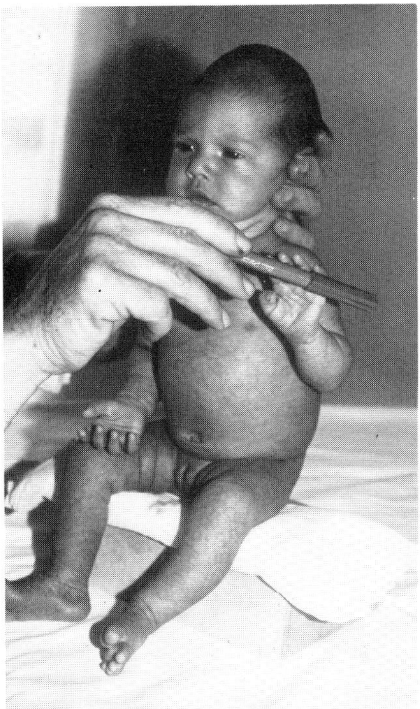

FIG. 89. Liberated motor activity: Second observational situation (J12). Infant grasps object, but releases this hold when object is lifted. Other hand is extended.

then try to recapture the infant's visual attention. An assistant is seated directly in front of the infant (Fig. 87). The infant is not immobilized. Short, discrete balancing motions of the body are added to the short, slight, pistonlike movements of the neck and head. It is important to maintain strict alignment in the head and trunk during this part of the examination. However, this alignment will be broken at the end of the maneuver as a means of estimating the effect of head movements on the activity of the arms. Indeed, in this situation, the expression of the LMA is much richer and reminiscent of that of an older infant.

The infant is now completely alert: the eyes move about and the infant appears interested in faces and the environment.

The upper extremities may rest alongside the body or may be animated by small, low-amplitude movements. It is easy to lift the infant's arms without resistance. Subsequently, the arms may be dropped without stimulating any jerking movements.

The hands are open wide and often rest on the bench or on the examiner's arms (Fig. 88). At this point, the grasp reflex has disappeared. Even if a small object put into the palm should provoke a slight flexion of the fingers, this grasp is very weak. Were one to lift the object, the grasp would not be strong enough to counter gravity (Fig. 89). The Moro reflex and the tonic neck reflex are inhibited as well. Deflection or rotation of the head is easily tolerated and does not stimulate any motor activity in the upper extremities.

Although the lower extremities are also involved in this total relaxation, their involvement is somewhat delayed. Resistance to passive stretching becomes progressively weaker, especially in the adductor muscles. Some feeble straightening attempts may be present in the initial phases of the maneuver, but these disappear rapidly if sufficient head support is maintained.

New motor activity is also observed in the trunk. Although the trunk is weak initially and requires some anterior support, it will straighten progressively. After 5–10 min, the natural cyphosis will disappear (Fig. 90). If a hand is placed behind the head, it is possible to feel this straightening as the head pushes up. The examiner will note that increasingly less strength is required to maintain the vertical position and to prevent the infant from falling forward or backward. At this point, it is possible to explore the LMA planned for the third situation.

Infant Seated behind the Small Desk

A small desk is placed in front of the infant. The desktop reaches the infant's epigastric level; the infant remains seated on the bench. The examiner stands behind the infant, holding the skull from above and grasping the parietal prominence on either side (Fig. 91). Equilibrium is

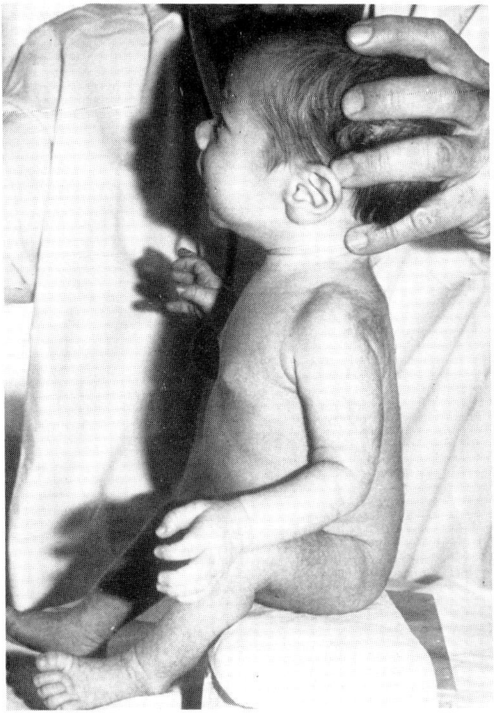

FIG. 90. Liberated motor activity: Second observational situation (J14). If infant is placed in sitting position, dorsal cyphosis will disappear after several minutes.

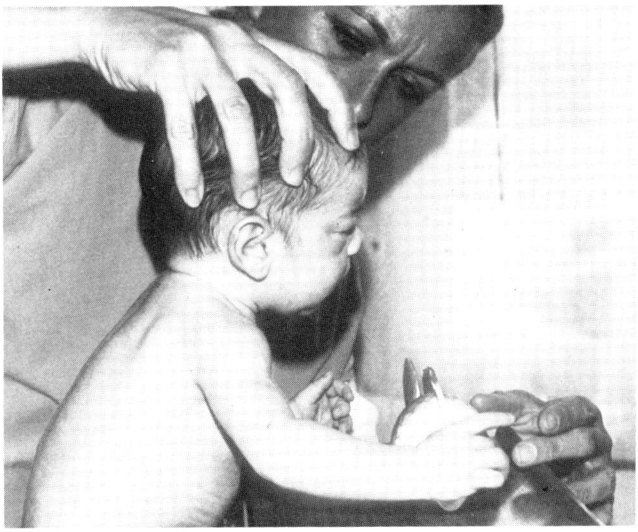

FIG. 91. Liberated motor activity: Third observational situation (J17). Examiner's hand has moved to vertex of skull. Infant does not use desk for support.

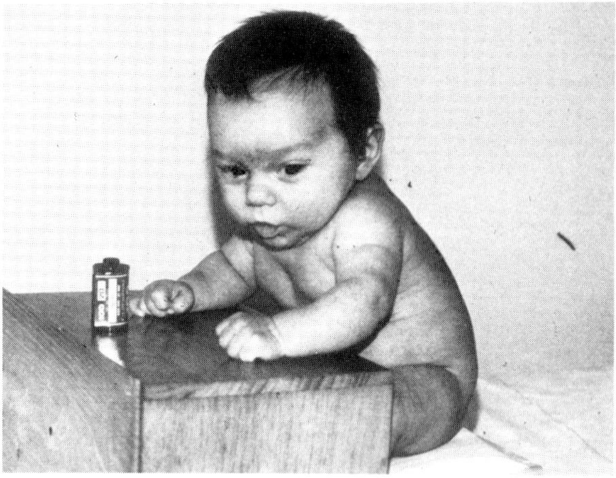

FIG. 92. Liberated motor activity: Third observational situation. Chronological age, 2 months; Corrected age, 1 month. Infant sits alone for several seconds.

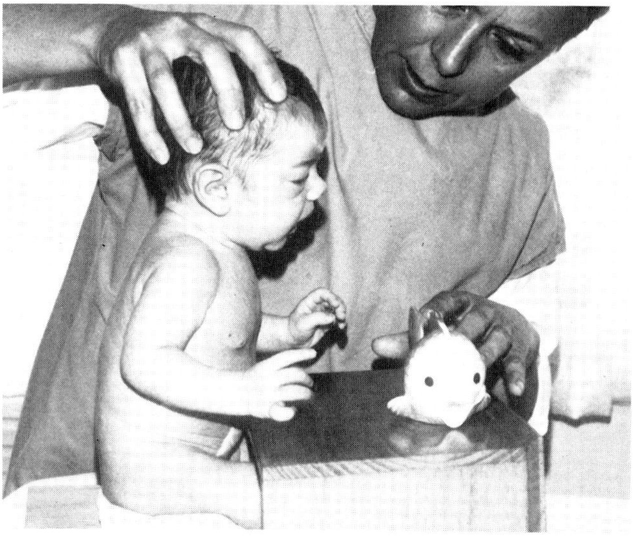

FIG. 93. Liberated motor activity: Third observational situation (J17). Object has caught infant's attention. Note position of examiner's hands.

established by supporting the infant's abdomen. The infant's position may be somewhat unstable at the beginning of this maneuver because of the different and decreased head support; however, it is possible for the infant to remain in this position without falling, even if all support is withdrawn for several seconds (Fig. 92). When this occurs, there is no obligatory motor response. Liberated motor activity persists and is manifest in the fol-

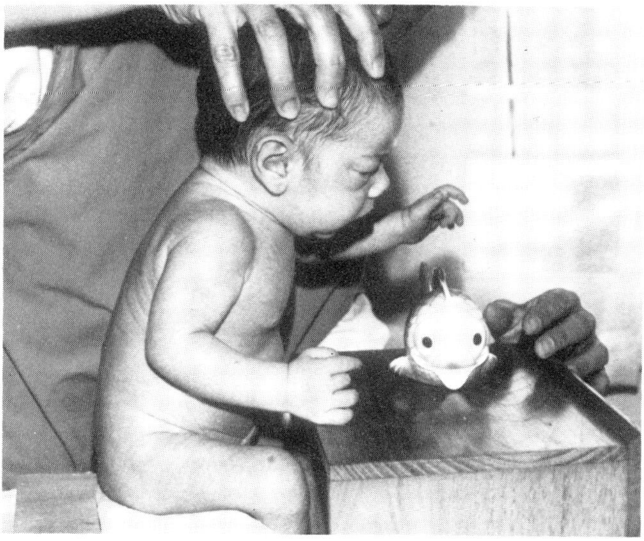

Fig. 94. Liberated motor activity: Third observational situation (J17). Infant becomes interested in this object and reaches toward it.

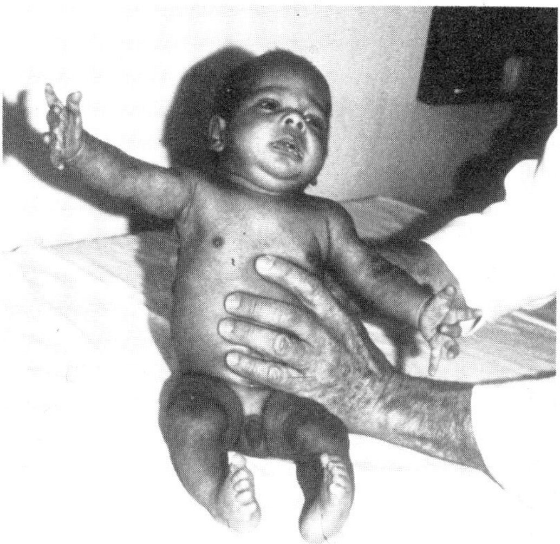

Fig. 95. Liberated motor activity: Precaution. If neck is not immobilized, head may be thrown backward abruptly.

lowing manner: the infant's attention shifts from the examiner to an object placed on the desk (Fig. 93). Once the infant becomes interested in the object, the hands will move toward it and may even grasp it (Fig. 94). These movements may be repeated as long as the infant remains attentive to the object. Postural tone of the trunk becomes even stronger during this maneuver. There is no postural collapse even if the examiner releases support to the infant's abdomen. Moreover, if the examiner withdraws support to the head, the position will be maintained for several seconds and the resulting drop of the head will only modify motor activity in the upper extremities.

Final Phase of the Examination

Certain of the previously described motor responses will persist for several minutes. The infant remains fascinated by the examiner and will visually follow his or her movement. Deflection of the neck will not initiate the Moro reflex and other responses are inhibited as well. Sudden noise does not provoke jerking and the grasping reflex is extinguished. The maneuver may be somewhat fatiguing and the trunk will not maintain this new tone. However, it is not uncommon for the infant to rest and relax without sleeping or crying.

Repetition of the Maneuver

Manual immobilization of the neck can be repeated without difficulty. These sessions contribute significantly to the rapidly strengthened postural regulation of the body. Uncontrolled and poorly inhibited head movements will be diminished as a consequence. It is possible to initiate LMA with the infant seated on the bench. Moreover, the examination can begin by studying the infant's behavior in relationship to an object on the desk.

Precautions

Approaching the Infant

It is important to avoid any external interferences or afferent stimuli which would provoke obligatory responses, thereby preventing liberated motor activity. The infant's comfort must be respected. For example, the room should be warm as the infant is naked during the examination. Newborns should be examined only after all vital signs have stabilized. Gastrointestinal distress may be an important obstacle. Postprandial distention or digestive difficulties will make the infant uncomfortable while seated. As a result, the infant may not cooperate with the examination. An older infant who has achieved postural head control will fight any attempt to immobilize the neck. Accordingly, infants should not be examined after this developmental milestone.

Immobilization of the Head and Neck

The examiner must grasp the infant's head firmly, but without causing undue discomfort. Hand position must be readjusted if the head begins to slip. All head movements must be prevented. These may be manifest in a number of ways. For example, the infant may throw the head backward in a straightening effort starting with the trunk, the hips, or the feet (Fig. 95). Conversely, the head may fall forward because of weak neck muscles (Fig. 96). The examiner must restrain efforts to push the neck backward and prevent the head from falling forward. Immobilization of the head will not preclude trunk movements that could create similar afferent stimuli. The examiner must maintain the head and neck in perfect alignment

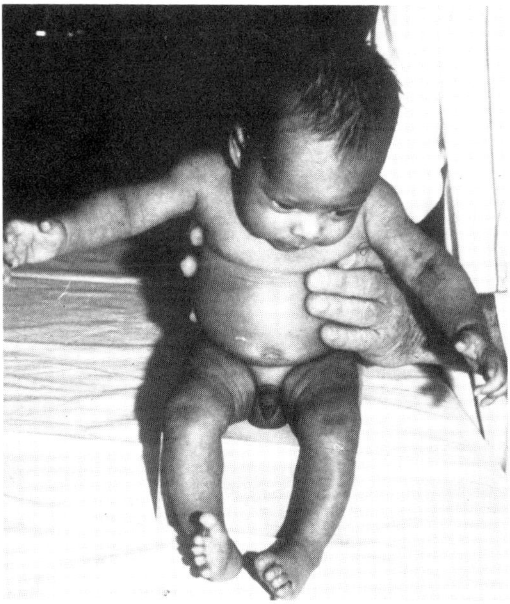

FIG. 96. Liberated motor activity: Precaution. If neck is not immobilized, head may fall forward.

in order to suppress this activity. Movements must be prevented even when the infant's position is changed. The goal of head and neck control differs in each of the three examination situations. While the infant is seated on the table, immobilization serves to inhibit obligatory motor activity rather than to provide support to the head. In this situation, the examiner holds the infant's neck firmly at the occipital region.

When the infant sits on the bench, head immobilization serves to strengthen postural tone of the trunk. The neck is not held directly; rather, the examiner grasps the posterior portion of the skull. In this instance, immobilization is important for head support rather than for inhibition of afferent stimuli, i.e., the examiner supports and directs the head only to the extent required by the maneuver.

Liberated motor activity becomes functional in the third examination situation in which the infant is placed behind the desk. The examiner holds the infant's skull at the vertex. There is no inhibitory role and man-

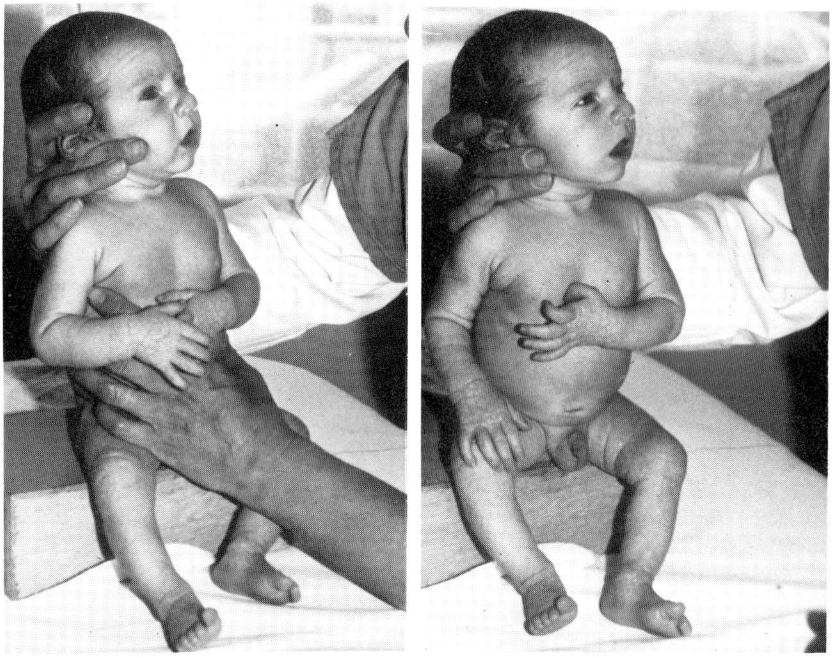

FIGS. 97 AND 98. Liberated motor activity: Precaution. Although abdominal counterbalance may be useful at start of maneuver, this support must be withdrawn later.

ual support is provided only as a safety precaution. The examiner may, in fact, release the head for relatively prolonged periods.

Countersupport of the Abdomen

Although abdominal support is not necessary, it is often quite useful at the beginning of the examination. This may be especially important if the infant's trunk is very weak. Abdominal support prevents falls that would disturb all motor activity. This support must be gentle, unobtrusive, and adapted to the changing examination situations (Figs. 97 and 98).

Infant Participation in the Examination

Maintaining the infant's involvement demands the constant attention of the examiner. The infant must be kept alert, but this must be accomplished without exaggerated stimulation that would be irritating.

The combination of visual, auditory, cutaneous, and proprioceptive stimuli represents a barrage of sensory input indispensable to the initiation and development of liberated motor activity. Communication with the infant becomes difficult or impossible in either of two situations. The infant may be very agitated and will not tolerate the sitting position. Should this occur, the examination must be interrupted. By contrast, the infant may remain calm but seem disinterested. In this event, the examiner should be patient in continuing the examination or should proceed to the third situation in which the infant usually performs as expected.

Examination Technique

The previously described precautions should be incorporated into the following description of the actual examination procedures. One initially approaches the infant by touching and stroking the body. Only then should the infant be placed on the examination table. If the infant resists the examination, he or she should be held and cuddled and then returned to the table. This comforting must be repeated until the necessary relaxation is achieved. This first step is often the most difficult. The examination will not be possible until this has been accomplished. Two difficult situations may present themselves–the infant resists immobilization or refuses to communicate, falling asleep.

The second observational situation is an intermediate but indispensible step in that it challenges expected motor effects. For example, motor inhibition must be maintained in order to achieve a complete but temporary extinction of the grasp and Moro reflexes. At the same time, the newly acquired motor activity must become increasingly apparent. This is especially important in the situation requiring the infant to be seated on the bench because there are no obstacles to interfere with motor activity in the upper extremities.

In the third situation, it becomes possible to analyze the strengths of postural tone in the neck and trunk. Because only minimal support is provided at the vertex and, optionally, at the abdomen, the infant will continuously adjust the posture to maintain the head and chest in an upright position. Sometimes, a voluntary motor activity in the upper extremities can be observed if the infant should become interested in a toy placed on the desk. Should this occur, observation of the liberated motor activity is complete. Such gestures should not be confused with random movements. To make this distinction, one must note both the movements of the hands and the infant's interest in the toy.

CLINICAL INDICATIONS

It is sometimes difficult to interpret results of the neuromotor examination. Evaluation of LMA is of particular interest in these instances. In addition, analysis of LMA is especially important in infants younger than 3 months who may exhibit inadequate alertness, hyperexcitability, incessant agitation, or hyperactive obligatory motor activity in response to minimal head movement. Moreover, we have found this evaluation useful in the analysis of motor anomalies of the upper extremities and the trunk, e.g., asymmetry, decreased motor activity, or abnormal motor response during movement of the extremities.

THEORETICAL IMPLICATIONS

Our study of LMA suggests that neuromotor expression typical of an older infant may actually underlie classic newborn behavior. It is therefore possible to describe two types of motor activity: 1) classic motor activity, composed of clustered reflexes, reaction postures, and obligatory

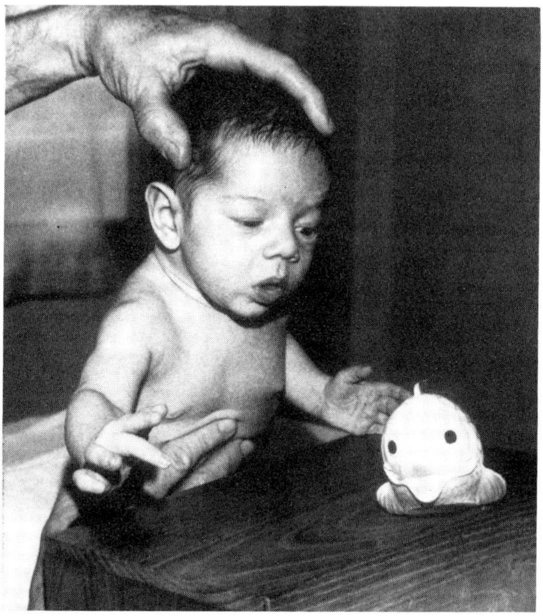

FIGS. 99, 100, 101, 102, AND 103. Liberated motor activity (J17). George sees toy fish. He reaches for tail of fish with his left hand. As he grasps fish, it flips over. George's astonishment and fascination are obvious.

motor responses generally controlled by the head and neck; and 2) liberated motor activity, apparent only if the classic motor activity is suppressed.

These two types of motor activity differ in that 1) head and neck control is absent in the classic situation; and 2) immobilization of the head

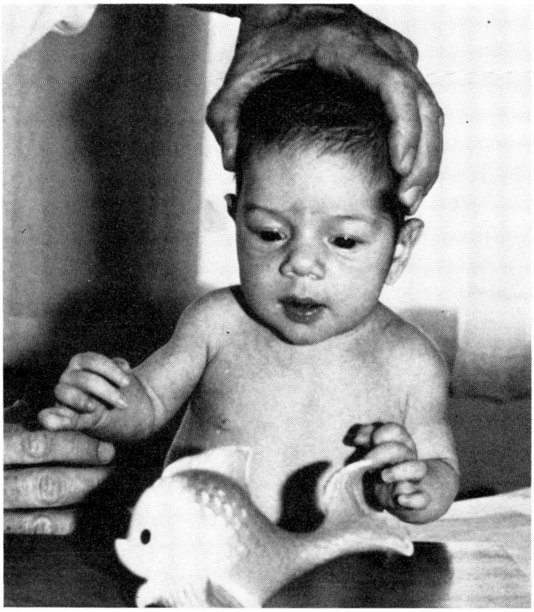

FIG. 100.

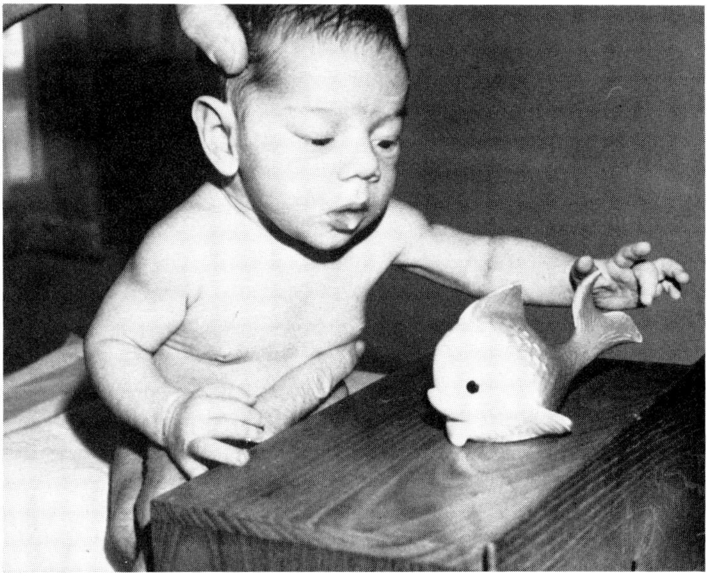

FIG. 101.

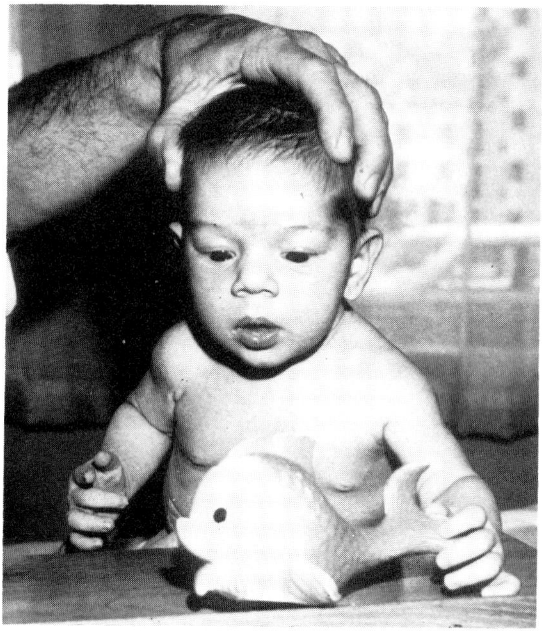

FIG. 102.

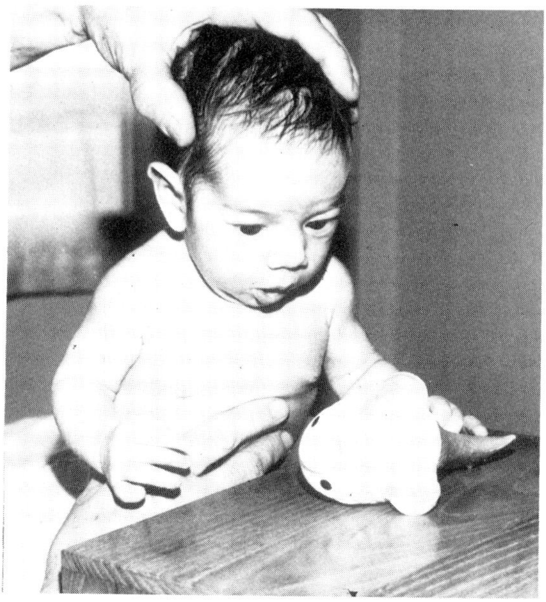

FIG. 103.

and neck is prerequisite to expression of liberated motor activity in the newly created situation.

Because of the subcortical origins of classic motor activity, it is expressed in universal reflexes, reactions, passive muscle tone, and obligatory motor responses. Accordingly, findings can be coded, compared across examinations, and recorded on preestablished developmental grids. This schematization contributes to the ease in executing and interpreting the neurological examination. Although the neurological examination does not explore the cerebral cortex, it should be possible to deduce from the findings either normal or abnormal cortical organization. Of course, an erroneous interpretation is possible, as demonstrated by an anencephalic infant who appears neurologically normal.

Because temporary suppression of all or most subcortical activities is prerequisite to expression of LMA, it would be invalid to use the classic reference system. The LMA demonstrates new motor responses that are not well understood and cannot be coded systematically at this time. Knowledge of LMA may be important in that these behaviors are similar to the motor activity found in older infants. LMA is therefore assumed to be of cortical origin.

As an example, we cite the motor activity observed in a 17-day-old infant photographed while sitting behind a desk grasping a toy that had caught his attention (Figs. 99–103). This example of very precocious motor regulation raises the issue of innate versus acquired learning. Research on neuroperception now in progress supports our hypothesis that a very high neurological organization is apparent in the newborn.

Appendices

RECORD FORM FOR MONTHLY EXAMINATION WITHIN THE FIRST YEAR

NAME SEX

DATE OF BIRTH

GESTATIONAL AGE ☐ WEEKS

CORRECTION FACTOR 40–G.A. = ☐ WEEKS

DATE	PRESENT AGE	CORRECTED AGE	EXAMINATION NUMBER	TESTED BY

HEAD CIRCUMFERENCE (see growth curves)

	1	2	3	4	5	6	7	8	9	10	11	12
cm												
+2 SD												
-2 SD												

ANTERIOR FONTANELLE

Normal												
Tense												
Depressed												

SUTURES

Normal												
Separated												
Overlapping												

USUAL PATTERN FOR WAKEFULNESS AND SLEEP

Normal												
Agitated, too much crying												
Lethargic, no crying												

ESTIMATION OF ALERTNESS DURING THE TEST

Satisfactory												
Constantly agitated												
Lethargic												

CRY

	1	2	3	4	5	6	7	8	9	10	11	12
Normal												
High-pitched												
Weak												
Monotonous												
Other												

SUCKING BEHAVIOR

	1	2	3	4	5	6	7	8	9	10	11	12
Normal												
Partial bottle-feeding												
No bottle-feeding												
Choking												

CONVULSIONS DURING THE PRECEDING MONTH

Absent												
Generalized												
Focal												
Febrile												
Infantile spasms												

HYPERTONIA OF ELEVATORS PALPEBRAE SUPERIORI

Absent												
Present												

SETTING-SUN SIGN

Absent												
Present												

MARKED STRABISMUS

Absent												
Present												

SUSTAINED NYSTAGMUS

Absent												
Present												

PURSUIT OF LIGHT

Present												
Absent												

ACOUSTIC BLINK REFLEX

Present												
Absent												
	1	2	3	4	5	6	7	8	9	10	11	12

ASYMMETRIC TONIC NECK REFLEX (POSTURAL)

	1	2	3	4	5	6	7	8	9	10	11	12
Normal pattern	tolerable			--- absent -			-------------			--- absent--		
Absent												
Present												

PERMANENT HYPERTONICITY OF NECK EXTENSORS

	1	2	3	4	5	6	7	8	9	10	11	12
Absent												
Present												

OPISTHOTONOS

	1	2	3	4	5	6	7	8	9	10	11	12
Absent												
Present												

CONSTANT CLOSURE OF THE HANDS

	1	2	3	4	5	6	7	8	9	10	11	12
Normal pattern	tolerable		no	----------		no	---------		no	--------		no-
Absent												
Present												
Thumb across the palm												

ASYMMETRY OF POSTURE OF LIMBS

	1	2	3	4	5	6	7	8	9	10	11	12
Absent												
Present												
Abnormal limb	indicate :											

FACIAL PARALYSIS right ☐ left ☐

	1	2	3	4	5	6	7	8	9	10	11	12
Absent												
Present												

SPONTANEOUS MOTOR ACTIVITY

	1	2	3	4	5	6	7	8	9	10	11	12
Low												
Medium = Normal												
High												
Asymmetric												
Repetitive												

ABNORMAL MOVEMENTS

	1	2	3	4	5	6	7	8	9	10	11	12
Absent												
Incessant Tremor												
Clonic movements												
Other												

DYSKINETIC MOVEMENTS OF THE LIMBS

Absent												
Present												
Abnormal limb	indicate :											

ADDUCTORS ANGLE

	40° to 80°			70° to 110°			100° to 140°			130° to 150°		
Normal pattern	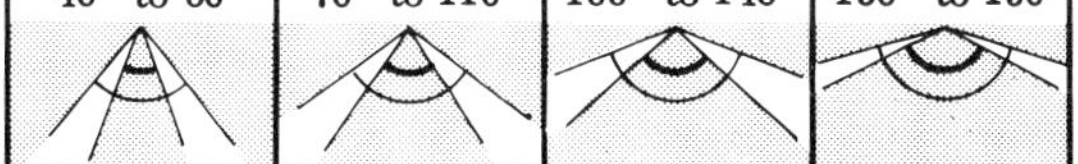											
Angle R + L												
Limited												
Exaggerated												
More limited right												
More limited left												

HEEL TO EAR

		80° to 100°			90° to 130°			120° to 150°			140° to 170°		
Normal pattern		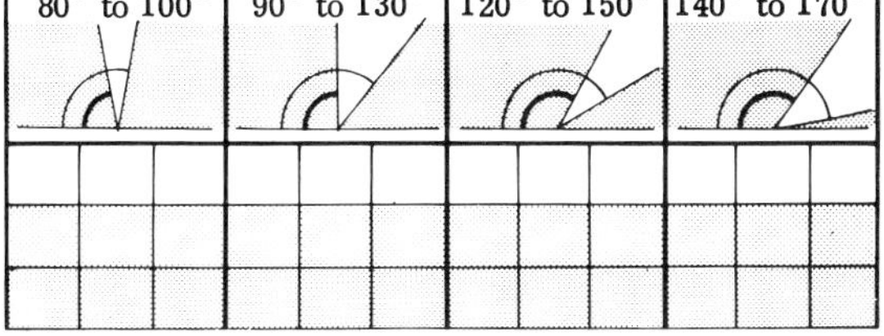											
Right	Angle												
	Limited												
	Exaggerated												
Left	Angle												
	Limited												
	Exaggerated												
		1	2	3	4	5	6	7	8	9	10	11	12
Excessive Hip Flexion													

POPLITEAL ANGLE

		1	2	3	4	5	6	7	8	9	10	11	12
Normal pattern		80° to 100°			90° to 120°			110° to 160°			150° to 170°		
Right	Angle												
	Limited												
	Exaggerated												
Left	Angle												
	Limited												
	Exaggerated												

DORSIFLEXION ANGLE OF THE FOOT

		1	2	3	4	5	6	7	8	9	10	11	12
Normal pattern		60° 70°			60° 70°			60° 70°			60° 70°		
Right	Angle (slow)												
	Angle (rapid)												
	"Slow" > 60°-70°												
	Difference "rapid-slow" > 10°												
Left	Angle (slow)												
	Angle (rapid)												
	"Slow" > 60°-70°												
	Difference "rapid-slow" > 10°												

	1	2	3	4	5	6	7	8	9	10	11	12
ASYMMETRY Right/left												

RESPONSE TO STRETCH

Jerky or Phasic												
Tonic												

SCARF SIGN

Normal pattern

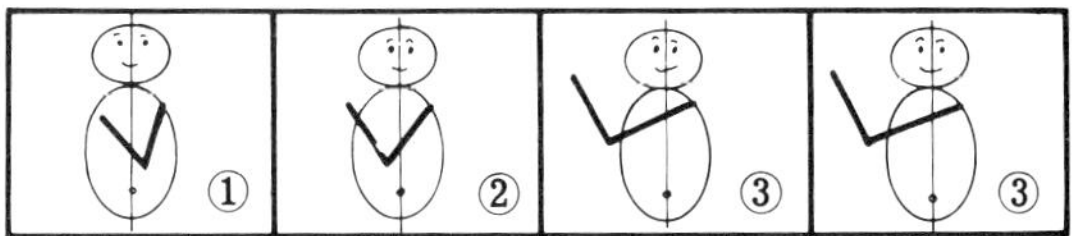

		1	2	3	4	5	6	7	8	9	10	11	12
Right	Position												
	Limited												
	Exaggerated												
Left	Position												
	Limited												
	Exaggerated												
ASYMMETRY	Right/left												

THE NEXT FOUR ITEMS WILL BE TESTED ONLY IF ASYMMETRY HAS BEEN OBSERVED BY THE MANEUVERS DESCRIBED ABOVE.

		1	2	3	4	5	6	7	8	9	10	11	12
FLAPPING OF THE FOOT	More ample right												
	More ample left												
SQUARE WINDOW	Angle smaller right												
	Angle smaller left												
FLAPPING OF THE HAND	More ample right												
	More ample left												
LATERAL ROTATION OF THE HEAD	More limited toward right												
	More limited toward left												

REPEATED VENTRAL FLEXION OF THE HEAD

	1	2	3	4	5	6	7	8	9	10	11	12
Identical												
More stiffness												

VENTRAL FLEXION OF THE TRUNK

	1	2	3	4	5	6	7	8	9	10	11	12
Normal (slight)												
Exaggerated												
Impossible												

DORSAL EXTENSION OF THE TRUNK

	1	2	3	4	5	6	7	8	9	10	11	12
Normal (impossible)												
Exaggerated												

LATERAL FLEXION OF THE TRUNK (tested only if an asymmetry R/L already detected)

	1	2	3	4	5	6	7	8	9	10	11	12
Normal												
Exaggerated												
More limited toward right												
More limited toward left												

ACTIVE CONTRACTION OF NECK FLEXORS

	1	2	3	4	5	6	7	8	9	10	11	12
Normal												
Difficult												
Absent (Passive)												
1) Impossible												

ACTIVE CONTRACTION OF NECK EXTENSORS

	1	2	3	4	5	6	7	8	9	10	11	12
Normal												
Difficult												
Absent (Passive)												
2) "Too Good"												

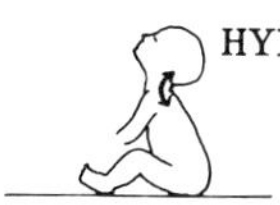

HYPERTONICITY OF NECK EXTENSORS

	1	2	3	4	5	6	7	8	9	10	11	12
Combination 1 + 2												

HEAD CONTROL

	1	2	3	4	5	6	7	8	9	10	11	12
Normal Pattern	absent	inconstant			--------- present ----------							
Present												
Absent												

PULLS TO SITTING POSITION

	1	2	3	4	5	6	7	8	9	10	11	12
Normal pattern	absent				inconstant			present				
Present												
Absent												

SITS ALONE MOMENTARILY

	1	2	3	4	5	6	7	8	9	10	11	12
Normal pattern	absent				inconstant			present				
Present												
Collapses forward												
Falls backward												

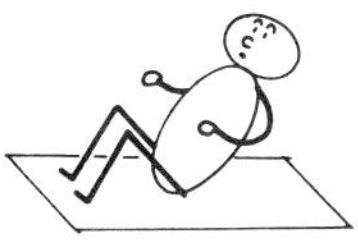

SITS ALONE 30 SECONDS OR MORE

	1	2	3	4	5	6	7	8	9	10	11	12
Normal pattern	absent					inconstant			present			
Present												
Absent												

STRAIGHTENING WITH LOWER LIMBS AND TRUNK (supporting reaction)

	1	2	3	4	5	6	7	8	9	10	11	12
Normal pattern	Present		incon-stant		-absent		---	Possible not sustained		Present		
Present												
Absent												
Scissoring												
Trunk arching												

AUTOMATIC WALKING

	1	2	3	4	5	6	7	8	9	10	11	12
Normal pattern	present			inconstant		------- absent ----------						
Present												
Absent												

PALMAR GRASP

Normal pattern	present		inconstant		---------- absent -----------							
Present												
Absent												
Asymmetry R/L												

RESPONSE TO TRACTION

Normal pattern	present		inconstant		---------- absent -----------							
Present												
Absent												
Asymmetry R/L												

MORO REFLEX

Normal pattern	present			inconstant		--------- absent --------						
Present												
Absent												
Asymmetry R/L												
Clonic movements + low threshold												

ABNORMAL LIMB IN THE LAST 4 MANEUVERS

☐ Right ☐ Left

ASYMMETRIC TONIC NECK REFLEX (evoked)

1	2	3	4	5	6	7	8	9	10	11	12

BICEPS REFLEX

		1	2	3	4	5	6	7	8	9	10	11	12
Right	Normal												
	Absent												
	Exaggerated												
Left	Normal												
	Absent												
	Exaggerated												
ASYMMETRY R/L													

ANKLE CLONUS

Absent												
Present right												
Present left												

KNEE JERK

Right	Normal												
	Absent												
	Exaggerated												
Left	Normal												
	Absent												
	Exaggerated												
ASYMMETRY R/L													
		1	2	3	4	5	6	7	8	9	10	11	12

LATERAL PROPPING REACTION

	1	2	3	4	5	6	7	8	9	10	11	12
Normal pattern	-- absent ---			-- absent ---			incon- stant		---	-- present -		
Present												
Absent												
Asymmetry R/L												

PARACHUTE

	1	2	3	4	5	6	7	8	9	10	11	12
Normal pattern	-- absent ---			-- absent ---			---	incon- stant		-- present -		
Present												
Absent												
Asymmetry R/L												

Abnormal limb in the last 2 maneuvers ☐ right ☐ left

CLINICAL IMPRESSION DURING THE FIRST YEAR

	1 - 3	4 - 6	7 - 9	10-12
MICROCEPHALUS intra-uterine post-natal				
HYDROCEPHALUS intra-uterine post-natal				
HYPEREXCITABILITY (irritable, restless sleep pattern, abnormal movements, low threshold for primary reflexes, upper eyelid hypertonia, persistent fisting).				
LETHARGY (sleepy and difficult to waken, reduced spontaneous movements, infrequent crying, poor or absent primary reflexes).				
ABNORMALITIES OF PASSIVE TONE 1) Global hypotonia ("floppy baby", trunk and limbs).				
2) Upper body hypotonia (weak neck flexion, exaggerated scarf sign, poor response to traction).				
3) Flexion hypertonia of lower limbs (persistence of neonatal angles, adductor, heel to ear, popliteal).				
4) Flexion hypertonia of upper limbs (persistent fisting and limited scarf sign).				
5) Imbalance in passive tone of trunk (reduced ventral flexion + increased dorsal extension).				
6) Asymmetric tone (hemisyndrome)				

Months

ABNORMALITIES OF ACTIVE TONE 1) Hyperactivity of neck extensors (head unable to drop forward).				
2) Hyperactivity of neck and trunk extensors (arching)				
3) Poor active tone, "floppy baby" (no head control, no sitting position, no standing position - according to normal pattern).				
PERIPHERAL NERVE PALSY face limbs				
DELAYED APPEARANCE OF POSTURAL REACTIONS (lateral propping and parachute).				
IMPAIRED HEARING				
STRABISMUS				
OTHER OCULAR ABNORMALITIES				
DEVELOPMENTAL DELAY (test or subtest).				
SEIZURES febrile nonfebrile				
EEG ABNORMALITY				
	1 - 3	4 - 6	7 - 9	10-12

Months

Name

Date of Birth

G.A.

Birthweight

SUMMARY AT THE END OF THE FIRST YEAR

NO ABNORMALITY

PATTERNS OF TRANSIENT ABNORMALITIES

1) Hyperexcitability
Hypertonia of neck extensors ☐

2) Hypotonia. Lethargy
Primary reflexes poor or absent ☐

3) Mimicking spastic diplegia ☐
(no relaxation in lower limbs, poor active tone, persisting primary reflexes, phasic contraction to stretch, exaggerated deep tendon reflexes).

4) Mimicking spastic hemiplegia ☐
(no relaxation on one side, asymmetric movements, exaggerated deep tendon reflexes).

5) Mimicking spastic quadriplegia ☐

6) Developmental delay ☐
(global or subtest abnormality).

7) Miscellaneous ☐

PATTERNS OF PERSISTENT ABNORMALITIES

1) Cerebral palsy
- spastic diplegia ☐
- spastic hemiplegia ☐
- quadriplegia ☐
- choreoathetosis ☐

2) Microcephalus ☐

3) Hydrocephalus ☐

4) Mental retardation ☐

5) Convulsions
- febrile ☐
- nonfebrile ☐

6) Sensory problems
- auditory ☐
- visual ☐

7) Miscellaneous ☐

ETIOLOGY

Genetic		Perinatal			
certain	☐	pre-natal	☐	Miscellaneous	☐
probable	☐	intra-partum	☐	Unknown	☐
		post-natal	☐		

References

1. Ajuriaguerra de J. Neuropsychologie du développement. Extrait de *l'Annuaire du Collège de France,* 1978, 379.
2. Amiel-Tison C. A method for neurologic evaluation within the first year of life. *In: Current Problems in Pediatrics.* Year Book Medical Publishers, Chicago, 1976, *VII*, n° 1.
3. Amiel-Tison C., Korobkin R. and Esque-Vaucouloux M.T. Neck extensor hypertonia: a clinical sign of insult to the central nervous system of the newborn. *Early Human Dev.*, 1977, *1*, 181.
4. Amiel-Tison C. A method for neurological evaluation within the first year of life: experience with full-term newborn infants with birth injury. *In: Major Mental Handicap: Methods and Costs of Prevention.* Ciba Foundation Symposium, no. 59. Elsevier, New York, 1978, p. 107.
5. Banker B. Q. and Larroche J. Cl. Periventricular leukomalicia of infancy. *Arch. Neurol. Psychiatr.*, 1962, *7*, 386.
6. Bayley N. *Bayley Scales for Infant Development.* The Psychological Corporation, New York, N.Y., 1969.
7. Bergström K. and Bille B. Computed tomography of the brain in children with minimal brain damage: a preliminary study of 46 children. *Neuropädiatrie,* 1978, *9*, 378.
8. Brunet O. and Lezine I. *Le développement psychologique de la première enfance.* 2e éd., Paris, Presses Universitaires de France, 1966.
9. Cockburn F. Discussion. *In: Ciba Foundation Symposium,* no. 59. Elsevier, 1978, p. 121.
10. Drillien C. M. Abnormal neurologic signs in the first year of life in low birth weight infants. Possible prognostic significance. *Dev. Med. Child. Neurol.*, 1972, *14*, 575.
11. Drillien C. M. Discussion. *In: Ciba Foundation Symposium,* no. 59. Elsevier, New York, 1978, p. 120.
12. Fitzhardinge P. and Pape K. E. Present status of the very low birth weight infant treated in a referral neonatal intensive care unit in 1974. *In: The Cost of Preventing Major Mental Handicap.* Ciba Foundation Symposium, no. 59. Elsevier, New York, 1978, p. 139.
13. Gesell A. and Amatruda C. S. *Developmental diagnosis: normal and abnormal child development.* Hoeber, New York, 1941.
14. Grenier A. Introduction à la journée d'études de dépistage et de traitement précoce des infirmes moteurs cérébraux. *Cahiers du cercle de documentation et d'information pour la rééducation des I.M.C.* Paris, 1972, *52*, 5.
15. Grenier A., Vima Ph., Solomiac J. and Solomiac J. Examen neuro-moteur complémentaire chez les nourrissons suspects d'I.M.C. *Cahiers du cercle de documentation et d'information pour la rééducation des I.M.C.*, Paris, 1975, *65*, 7.
16. Grenier A. La Réaction Latérale d'Abduction chez les nourrissons à risque élevé. Société de Neurologie Infantile. *Congrès de Marseille,* 1977, p. 69.
17. Hirsch J. F., Lacombe A., Pierre-Kahn A. and Renier D. Mesure de la pression intracrânienne par palpeur de fontanelle. *Neurochirurgie,* 1978, *24*, 89.

18. Illingworth R. S. *The Development of the Infant and Young Child,* 5th ed. Churchill Livingstone, London, 1972, p. 377.

19. Koupernik C. and Dailly R. *Development neuro-psychique du nourrisson,* 3ᵉ éd., Presses Universitaires de France, Paris, 1976.

20. Lalande J., Le Loc'h H. and Doyon H. Enquête sur le devenir des nouveau-nés traités en Centre de Soins Intensifs. III Les anomalies neurologiques. *Arch. Fr. Pédiatr.*, 1978, *35*, 351.

21. Le Métayer M. Bilan neuromoteur du nourrisson normal ou pathologique. *Cahiers du Cercle de documentation et d'information pour la rééducation des I.M.C.*, Paris, 1973, *54*, 3.

22. Le Métayer M. Bilan neuromoteur du nourrisson normal et du nourrisson pathologique. *Cahiers du cercle de documentation et d'information pour la rééducation des I.M.C.*, Paris, 1975, *65*, 35.

23. Micheli J. L. Discussion. *In: Ciba Foundation Symposium,* no. 59. Elsevier, New York, 1978, p. 123.

24. Minkowski A., Amiel-Tison Cl., Cukier F., Dreyfus-Brisac C., Relier J. P. and de Bethmann O. Long term follow-up and sequelae of asphyxiated infants. In: *Intrauterine Asphyxia and the Developing Fetal Brain.* Year Book Medical Publishers, Chicago, 1977, p. 309.

25. Nelhaus G. Composite international and interracial graphs. *Pediatrics,* 1968, *41*, 106.

26. Prechtl H. F. R. and Beintema D. The neurological examination of fullterm newborn infant. *Clinics in Developmental Medicine* no. 12. Spastics International Medical Publications, London, 1964, p. 74.

27. Prechtl H. F. R. Assessment and significance of behavioural states. In: *Brain, Fetal and infants.* S.R. Berenberg, Ed. Martinus Nijhoff Medical Division, The, Hague, 1977, p. 79.

28. Saint-Anne Dargassies S. *Le développement neurologique du nouveau-né à terme et prématuré.* Masson, Paris, 1974, p. 337.

29. Stambak M. and Ajuriaguerra de J. Evolution de l'estensibilité musculaire depuis la naissance jusqu'á l'âge de 2 ans. *Presse Médicale,* 1958, *66*, 24.

30. Stewart A., Turcan D., Rawlings G., Hart S. and Gregory S. Outcome for infants at high resk of major handicap In *The Cost of Preventing Major Mental Handicap.* Ciba Foundation Symposium, no. 50. Elsevier, New York, 1978, p. 151.

31. Tabary J. C. Elements de psychologie. *Editions Médicales et Universitaires.* Paris, 1978, p. 475.

32. Tardieu G. Infirmités motrices cérébrales. *Rev. Neuropsychiatr. Infantile,* 1968, *1-2*, 1.

33. Tardieu G. and Lagert P. Le tonus et ses troubles en clinique. *Encycl. Med. Chir. Paris, Système nerveux,* 4.2.02., 17 007 A20.

34. Thomas A. and Ajuriaguerra de J. *Etude sémiologique du tonus musculaire.* Editions Medicales Flammarion, Paris, 1949.

35. Thomas A. and Saint-Anne Dargassies S. *Etudes neurologiques sur le nouveau-né et le jeune nourrisson.* Masson, Paris 1952, pp. 434.

36. Touwen B. Neurological development in infancy. *Clinics in Developmental Medicine* no. 58. Spastics International Medical Publications. London, 1976, pp. 150.

37. Vojta V. *Die cerebralen Feoeegungsstarungen in Saüglinglingsalter.* F. Enke Verlag, Stuttgart, 1974.

38. Vyhmeister N., Schneider S. and Cha C. Cranial transillumination norms of premature infant. *J. Pediatrics,* 1977, *91*, 980.

39. Wealthall S. R. and Smallwood R. Methods of measuring intracranial pressure via the fontanelle without puncture. *J. Neurol. Neurosurg. Psychiatry,* 1974, *37,* 88.

40. Gagnard L. and Le Metayer M. Rééducation des infirmes moteurs cérébraux. *Expansion Scientifique Française.* Paris, *1,* 1979, p. 140.

INDEX

Abduction of the hip, 61
Acoustic blink reflex, 15
Active tone, 2, 3, 30
Adductors angle, 19
Ankle clonus, 43
Arteriovenous malformation, 7
Asymmetric tonic neck reflex, 15, 16, 41
Asymmetry, 17
Auscultation of the scalp, 7
Automatic walking, 39
Axial alignment, 62

Biceps reflex, 43
Brachycephaly, 7
Bruit, 7

Cerebral atrophy, 7
Classification, 50
Clinical significance, 84
Clonic movements, 18
Clonus, 27
Closure of the hands, 17
Comprehension, 8
Contraction of neck extensors, 32
Coronal suture, 5
Craniostenosis, 5
Cry, 13

Deep tendon reflexes, 43
Demonstration, 89
Directed motor activity, 57
Dolichocephaly, 7
Dorsiflexion angle of the foot, 22, 23

Emotional reaction, 8
Extension of the trunk, 30
Extensor muscles of the neck, 16
 of the trunk, 49

Facial paralysis, 17
Fencing position, 15, 16
First trimester, 50
First year, 50
Flapping feet, 24, 27
Flapping maneuver, 2
Flapping of the hands, 26, 27
Flexion of hands, 25
 of trunk, 2
Fontanelles, 5, 12

Grid, use of critique, 45

Handicap score, 54
Head circumference, 5, 12
 charts, 6
 curve, 7
Head control, 33
Heel to ear, 22
Heel to ear angle, 20
Hydranencephaly, 7
Hydrocephaly, 5, 7
Hyperflexion of the hips, 22
Hypertonia of elevators palpebrae superiori, 13
 of neck extensors, 15
Hypertonicity, 49
 of the spinal muscles, 38

Indications, 81
Induction, 76

of lateral abduction reaction, 77–80
Interobserver reliability, 48

Knee jerk, 43

Labile stiffening, 18
Landau reflex, 2, 3
Lateral abduction reaction, 57, 59–81, 84
Lateral flexion of the head, 64
of the trunk, 29, 30
Lateral propping reaction, 44, 45
Lateral rotation of the head, 2, 27
Leukomalacia, 55
Level of alertness, 8
Liberated motor activity, 87–97, 99, 100, 101, 103, 104, 106–108
LMA, 106, 109
analysis, 105
evaluation, 105
Locomotion, 3

Moro reflex, 41, 42
Motor anomalies, transient, 53
Motor development, 8

Neck extensors, 32, 49
Neck flexor muscles, 49
Neck flexors, 31
Neuromotor anomolies, 52
Nystagmus, 14

Opisthotonos, 16

Palmar grasp, 39, 40
Parachute maneuver, 44
Parachute reaction, 45
Passive tone, 1, 19
of the spinal axis, 29
Phasic contraction, 23
Popliteal angle, 21, 22
Porencephaly, 7
Positive transillumination, 7
Postural attitude, 3
Postural reactions, 38
Posture of limbs, 17
Primary reflexes, 38, 39
Psychomotor assessment, 8
Pull-to-sitting, 31, 34
Pursuit of light, 14

Response to traction, 41
Resting tone, 2
Risk conditions, 81

Scarf sign, 2, 24, 25
School age difficulties, 53
Second and third trimesters, 51
Sensory perception, 8
Setting sun sign, 14
Sitting, 35, 36
Sleep patterns, 13
Social factors, 8
Spinal muscles, 37
Spontaneous motor activity, 18
Square window, 27
State, 68
Strabismus, 14
Straightening, 36, 37
of the trunk, 37
reaction, 37
with neck flexors, 31
Subdural effusion, 7
Subdural hematoma, 85
Sucking, 13
Sutures, 5
Suture synostosis, 5
Suture width, 12
Swallowing, 13

Tendon reflexes, 38
Tonic contraction, 23
Transillumination, 7
Tremors, 18

Ventral flexion of the head, 27, 29
of the trunk, 28, 29
Ventral suspension, 45
Vestibular and visual postural reactions, 43